CALCULATION SKILLS
FOR NURSES

Student Survival Skills Series

Survive your nursing course with these essential guides for all student nurses:

Medicine Management Skills for Nurses, 2nd Edition
Claire Boyd
9781119807926

Clinical Skills for Nurses
Claire Boyd
9781118448779

Study Skills for Nurses
Claire Boyd
9781118657430

Care Skills for Nurses
Claire Boyd
9781118657386

Communication Skills for Nurses
Claire Boyd and Janet Dare
9781118767528

CALCULATION SKILLS
FOR NURSES

Second Edition

Claire Boyd

RGN, Cert Ed
Practice Development Trainer

WILEY Blackwell

This edition first published 2022
© 2022 John Wiley & Sons Ltd

Edition History
First Edition (2013)

Registered Office(s)
John Wiley & Sons, Inc., 111 River Street, Hoboken, NJ 07030, USA
John Wiley & Sons Ltd, The Atrium, Southern Gate, Chichester, West Sussex, PO19 8SQ, UK

Editorial Office
9600 Garsington Road, Oxford, OX4 2DQ, UK

For details of our global editorial offices, customer services, and more information about Wiley products visit us at www.wiley.com.

Wiley also publishes its books in a variety of electronic formats and by print-on-demand. Some content that appears in standard print versions of this book may not be available in other formats.

Library of Congress Cataloging-in-Publication Data Applied for

PB [9781119808121]

Cover Design: Wiley
Cover Image: © chuwy/Getty Images, © rambo182/Getty Images

Set in 9/12pt TradeGothic by Straive, Pondicherry, India

Printed in Singapore
M000922_210722

Contents

Part 3: Putting it All Into Practice 119

Part 4: Testing Your Knowledge 191

Part 5: Appendices 225

Preface

This book is the second edition and continues to be designed to assist ALL student healthcare workers in the field of calculations. It has also proved helpful for qualified healthcare professionals needing a little more practice and confidence. All exercises are related to practice and the healthcare environment. Chapter 1 incorporates a pre-assessment quiz to identify any areas needing to be revisited. Chapters 2 and 3 take the reader through the maths basics. The book then goes through the 'bread and butter' of everyday calculations used on a daily basis in health care.

The book incorporates many activities to check understanding, and is laid out in a simple to follow step-by-step approach. It ends with Knowledge tests that relate everything the reader has learned, to practice situations. The book also incorporates an example of Employment Services calculations test papers, as newly-qualified students and new healthcare employees are often asked to complete a calculations test when being interviewed for a job. All answers can be located at the back of the book.

The aim of this book is to start the individual on a journey through many healthcare-related exercises in order to build confidence and competence. It has been compiled using quotes and tips from student nurses themselves; it is a book by students for students.

Claire Boyd
Bristol

Introduction

Hello, my name is Claire.

This is the second edition of a book written with the assistance of nursing students, informing me of what they wanted included in a book to help them with their nursing calculations.

I have been a Practice Development Trainer in a large NHS Trust for many years and a nurse for over 30 years. It has been my pleasure to teach literally thousands of students in a variety of healthcare related subjects including my favourite subject – nursing calculations. I know that not all of you share my passion, some have even told me that they feel physically sick at the mention of the word 'mathematics' and have expressed a fear of making a calculations error in drug administration and also taking a calculations test. Fear not, I will take you by the hand and lead you through the streets of London (opps! Sorry that was a song) and lead you through some basic maths revision, leading on to more complex calculations and on to those dreaded maths tests. I think I am best placed to prepare you for the tests as I actually write many of them!

Nursing has certainly evolved since the first addition of this book, not least the development of the Nursing Associate. You will see many Glossary terms, such as the following one explaining the role of these highly skilled healthcare professionals.

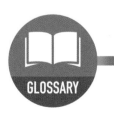

GLOSSARY

Nursing Associate
The Nursing Associate is a member of the multidisciplinary nursing team in England that aims to bridge the gap between Health Care Assistants (HCA's) and Registered Nurses (RN's). Nursing Associates have been accepted onto the Nursing and Midwifery (NMC) register in England since January 2019.

You will also see directions to websites to assist the reader, at the bottom of the chapter pages, like these ones:

USEFUL WEB RESOURCES:

www.nmc.org.uk
www.skillsforhealth.org.uk

This book came into fruition by listening to student nurses – their wants and needs. This second edition has included a wider audience Nursing Associates, Overseas nurses and many more, and I have been grateful for the reviews from students and other readers who have given me suggestions for improvements for the new edition:

1. More practice activities – tick
2. Title change for more inclusivity – tick
3. More test questions – tick
4. More on looking at budgets and interpreting data – tick
5. Pointers to websites – tick

There are test questions for student nurses, newly qualified nurses, nurse associates, nursing assistants, paediatric nurses, midwives, mental health nurses, learning disabilities nurses, and the nurse prescriber (NMP).

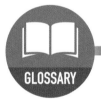

GLOSSARY

Nurse Prescriber
Post graduate nurses who have been licensed to issue medications to patients without a doctor being present or assessing the patient. Also known as Non-Medical Prescribing Nurse (NMP)

There are also many more exercises and activities to get stuck into, and examples whereby you will see a box like this:

Let me show you an example...

1   If you buy a rooster for the purpose of laying eggs and you expect to get 3 eggs each day for breakfast, how many eggs will you have after three weeks?

ANSWER: $3 \times 7 = 21$
$3 \times 7 = 21$
$3 \times 7 = 21$ TOTAL = 63 Eggs

WRONG!
Roosters are male chickens and don't lay eggs! D'oh!

OK, so that was a bit of fun! Don't worry if you got fooled by this trick question, I did too when I first saw it. I just wanted to show you that we all make mistakes, but if we take our time, and work through any question methodically, we can work it out. After all, the majority of healthcare questions just rely on your ability to **add, subtract, divide** or **multiply** – yes, it really is that simple!

This book is divided into four parts:

Part 1: Diagnosis – includes assessing your own ability and basic revision. You can miss out these chapters if you feel you don't need to work through them but this will give you a good grounding in basic maths, preparing you for the more complex questions.

Part 2: Understanding nursing calculations – this will show you what you need to know in the clinical area, such as working out drug dosages.

Part 3: Putting it all into practice – this will show you where the calculations we have worked through are applied in practice. It will show us that mathematics is used in many different areas in health care, including undertaking sample test questions, and working with budgets.

Part 4: Testing your knowledge and understanding – this is where we can monitor our increased abilities and showing us our progress.

I will show you how I approach maths problems: I believe firmly in using formulas for working out drug dosages, but I am aware that an understanding of how these formulas work must first be established, and a rough estimate of the correct answer should always be at the back of our minds. It is for this reason that I have produced the formulas in a handy format on the inside back cover for you to photocopy and laminate (for infection control, to be wiped clean) and keep in your pocket.

This book has been related to the **NMC Standards** for nursing and midwifery education (May 2018), Proficiency for registered nurses (May 2018), Proficiency for Nursing Associates (October 2018), Pre-registration Nursing Associate programme (October 2018) and The Code – Professional Standards for practice and behaviour for nurses, midwives and nursing associates (October 2018) and the NMC Essential Skills Clusters. However, this book is designed to assist anyone working in the healthcare setting requiring mathematical assistance.

In short, this book is designed to instil confidence and competence in the area of calculations to healthcare professionals. It is designed to be used as a building block, a platform for the rest of your healthcare career.

Acknowledgements

I, along with the publishers, would particularly like to thank all the nursing students who helped develop this book into what it is. Also, to the group of overseas nurses I met this year who told me that this series of books was on their reading list and they particularly liked the humour in it – thank you. Also, the student nurses who gave direction on what they also wanted included in this book and the other student healthcare professionals asking for more questions to do with their specific branch of healthcare – the Midwives, Paediatric Nurses and Mental Health Nurses, etc. – your wish is our command! Also, the Nursing Associates who wanted a book to bridge the gap between Nursing Assistants and Registered Nurses – again your wish is granted!

I would also like to extend my thanks to Magenta Styles (Associate Editorial Director) for her guidance and direction and to the team at Wiley-Blackwell for their support.

I dedicate this book to my loving family: husband Rob (for the use of his photographs), and to my grandson Owen who likes to play our favourite maths game with me – taking all the chocolates out of the tin and laying them out and counting them and making a couple disappear each time. Adding and subtraction is so much fun, Yum! Also, to baby Rhys who is right that Granny's notes are much more fun when scrunched up to make snowballs out of! Also, thanks to Simon, Louise and David for all their assistance in helping to develop the book series.

Latin Abbreviations

Here is a list of some Latin abbreviations that you may see on prescription forms:

AC	*ante cibum* **(before food)**
BD	*bis die* **(twice daily)**
OD	*omni die* **(every day)**
OM	*omni mane* **(every morning)**
ON	*omni nocte* **(every night)**
PC	*post cibum* **(after food)**
PRN	*pro re nata* **(when required)**
QDS	*quater die sumendus* **(to be taken four times daily)**
QQH	*quarta quaque hora* **(every 4 hours)**
STAT	**immediately**
TDS	*ter die sumendus* **(to be taken three times daily)**
TID	*ter in die* **(three times daily)**

THE 24-HOUR CLOCK

Time	24-hour clock	Can be expressed as
1 am	0100	01:00
2 am	0200	02:00
3 am	0300	03:00
4am	0400	04:00
5am	0500	05:00
6 am	0600	06:00
7 am	0700	07:00
8 am	0800	08:00
9 am	0900	09:00
10 am	1000	10:00
11 am	1100	11:00
12 mid-day	1200	12:00
1 pm	1300	13:00
2 pm	1400	14:00
3 pm	1500	15:00
4 pm	1600	16:00
5 pm	1700	17:00
6 pm	1800	18:00
7 pm	1900	19:00
8 pm	2000	20:00
9 pm	2100	21:00
10 pm	2200	22:00
11 pm	2300	23:00
12 mid-night	2400	24:00

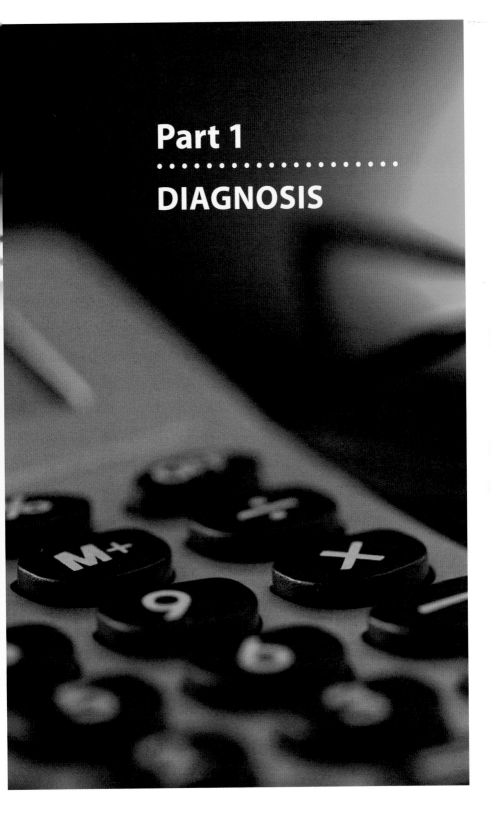

Part 1
. . . .
DIAGNOSIS

Chapter 1
· ·
CALCULATIONS
SELF-ASSESSMENT

Calculation Skills for Nurses, Second Edition. Claire Boyd.
© 2022 John Wiley & Sons Ltd. Published 2022 by John Wiley & Sons Ltd.

LEARNING OUTCOMES

By the end of this chapter you will have a better understanding of your strengths and weaknesses relating to calculations and which sections of the book you should focus on to improve your abilities.

To assess your own calculations ability, it is recommended that you complete the self-assessment in this chapter. It will help you to identify any area that you have difficulty with, and that you need to brush up on. You can use a calculator but first, why not have a go without one? This is because the NMC states that nurses should not rely too heavily on calculators. Attempting the self-assessment will also help you to identify your own improvement when you attempt the Knowledge Tests at the end of this book, where everything we have learned throughout the book gets put into practice. Don't worry if you don't answer everything correctly first time around: just go to Chapter 2 and Chapter 3 and work through the practice exercises.

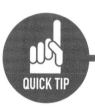

QUICK TIP

Remember the rule of 5s!

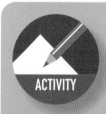

ACTIVITY

Activity 1.1

1   6.7 + 4.9 =
2   119 – 27 =
3   5.91 × 7.42 =
4   8 / 2.5 =

5	Round 0.78 to one decimal place.
6	Round 0.31 to one decimal place.
7	Round 4.72 to one decimal place.
8	Round 2.33 to one decimal place.
9	Round 9.45 to one decimal place.
10	Round 3.44 to one decimal place.
11	Round 2.418 to two decimal places.
12	Round 9.234 to two decimal places.
13	Round 0.915 to two decimal places.
14	Round 0.522 to two decimal places.
15	Round 2.340 to two decimal places.
16	Round 6.711 to two decimal places.
17	Round 0.8255 to three decimal places.
18	Round 1.5868 to three decimal places.
19	Change 39.4 to a whole number.
20	Change 31.7 to a whole number.
21	Change 39.9 to a whole number.

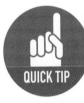

QUICK TIP

Remember: milligrams are *smaller* than grams.

22	Change 6000 mg into grams.
23	Change 0.7 micrograms into milligrams.
24	Change 9 micrograms into nanograms.

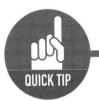

QUICK TIP

Remember: micrograms are *larger* than nanograms.

25 Change 0.03 g into milligrams.
26 Change 2.5 L into millilitres.

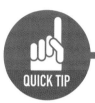

Remember: always make it clear if your answer has a decimal point.

27 Change 92 kg into grams.
28 Change 8 kg into grams.
29 Change 64.5 micrograms into milligrams.
30 Change 1527 micrograms into milligrams.
31 Change 0.02 mg into grams.
32 Change 1.2 mg into micrograms.
33 What is 25% of 500 mL?
34 What percentage is 92 of 150?
35 What is 10% of 233?
36 Change $\dfrac{4}{5}$ to a decimal with one decimal place.
37 Change $\dfrac{175}{5}$ to a decimal.
38 Change $\dfrac{1}{8}$ to a decimal with one decimal place.
39 How much stock solution is present in 200 mL of diluted solution if expressing this as a ratio of 1 in 5?
40 How much stock solution is present in 200 mL of diluted solution if expressing this as a ratio of 1:5?
41 How much stock solution is present in 600 mL of diluted solution if expressing this as a ratio of 1 in 3?
42 Write 60% as a fraction.
43 Write 0.75 as a percentage.
44 If you scored 90 out of 180 in a test, what percentage did you score?
45 Change 1 stone into kg.
46 Change 3 lb into kg.
47 Change 80 kg into pounds.

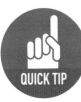

QUICK TIP

Remember: the mode is the most common figure in a set of figures.

48 What is the mode of 19, 19, 19.2, 20, 20.3 and 25?
49 What is the range of 6, 6.2, 9, 9.5 and 10?
50 What is the mean of 52, 52.4, 61, 67 and 70?

KEY POINT

- Understanding your own strengths and weaknesses in calculations.

USEFUL WEB RESOURCES

http://www.bbc.co.uk/schools/gcsebitesize/maths/number
www.mathcentre.ac.uk/students.php/health/arithmetric/
  rules/resources/

Chapter 2

CALCULATIONS REVISION

Calculation Skills for Nurses, Second Edition. Claire Boyd.
© 2022 John Wiley & Sons Ltd. Published 2022 by John Wiley & Sons Ltd.

LEARNING OUTCOMES

By the end of this chapter you will have familiarised yourself with maths basics and decimals, percentages, fractions, ratios and averages.

FEELING A BIT RUSTY?

Don't worry if picking up this book and the word 'calculations' gave you palpitations! We'll start nice and gently and summarise the basics. You may remember most of this already and feel confident enough to skip this chapter, and the next completely, or you may wish to build up your confidence and reacquaint yourself with the basics.

Symbols and Signs

+	plus or addition sign; example: **6 + 9 = 15**
−	decrease, subtract or minus sign; example: **11 − 4 = 7**
×	multiply or 'times by' sign; example: **9 × 6 = 54**
÷ or **/**	division or 'divide by' sign; example: **25/5 = 5**
=	the equals sign; example: **9 × 10 = 90**
:	Ratio
>	greater than
<	less than

Seeing this sign **/** means divided by. . .

ADDITION

Maths can be so much easier than you thought as a lot of the time we just need to use our adding skills. For example, a common nursing skill is to tot up a patient's fluid intake.

Let me show you an example. . .

Patient A's total oral intake of fluid has been:

Water 50 mL

Tea 150 mL

Water 150 mL

Tea 75 mL

Coffee 50 mL

Water 75 mL

Cola 200 mL

Cocoa 100 mL

All we need to do is add up all these figures:

$50 + 150 + 150 + 75 + 50 + 75 + 200 + 100 = 850$ mLs

To begin with, I did a quick rough mental calculation so I knew the answer would be 800 and something. So, 850 mLs looks about right. We will look at Fluid Charts in more detail in Chapter 12.

Sometimes, when we talk 'maths', this very word can make us quiver and we put up a brick wall and try to avoid the task in hand. But all we have to do is practice and look at the problem calmly and break the question down.

SUBTRACTION

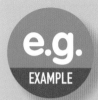

Let me show you an example. . .

A baby's nappy weighs 15 grams when dry. The nappy now weighs 123 grams. How much urine has the baby passed? **NOTE**: 1 gram = 1 mL.

ANSWER: This is a very simple subtraction question and all we have to do is subtract the weight of the dry nappy from the weight of the wet nappy: 123 grams – 15 grams = 108 mLs.

Have a go at doing one yourself to build your confidence.

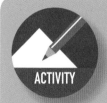

Activity 2.1

A baby's nappy weighs 18 grams when dry. The nappy now weighs 135 grams. How much urine has the baby passed? **NOTE**: 1 gram = 1 mL.

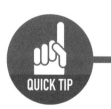

Don't over complicate the maths. Break everything down into bite-size pieces.

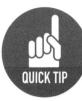

QUICK TIP

It is a good idea to reacquaint yourself with your times tables.

	1	2	3	4	5	6	7	8	9	10	11	12
1	1	2	3	4	5	6	7	8	9	10	11	12
2	2	4	6	8	10	12	14	16	18	20	22	24
3	3	6	9	12	15	18	21	24	27	30	33	36
4	4	8	12	16	20	24	28	32	36	40	44	48
5	5	10	15	20	25	30	35	40	45	50	55	60
6	6	12	18	24	30	36	42	48	54	60	66	72
7	7	14	21	28	35	42	49	56	63	70	77	84
8	8	16	24	32	40	48	56	64	72	80	88	96
9	9	18	27	36	45	54	63	72	81	90	99	108
10	10	20	30	40	50	60	70	80	90	100	110	120
11	11	22	33	44	55	66	77	88	99	110	121	132
12	12	24	36	48	60	72	84	96	108	120	132	144

MULTIPLICATION

Next, we have a very basic multiplication question. At first glance you may not notice how basic the question is:

A patient has been prescribed an inhaler due to their Chronic Obstructive Pulmonary Disease (COPD). The inhaler will need to last 28 days. The patient takes three inhalations daily from their inhaler device. How many inhalations does the patient take over the 28 days and will there be enough medication in the device for this period? **NOTE**: Inhaler contains 200 doses.

ANSWER:

3 = inhalations per day

28 = number of days required

3 × 28 = 84 doses

Therefore, the inhaler device has more than sufficient medication for this time period because it contains 200 doses and only 84 are required for this time period. There is therefore plenty to spare.

DIVISION

We can also work out some basic concentrations of medications in volume using division. Once you have been shown how to do it – it really is very simple! **NOTE**: we will be looking at slightly more complicated percentage concentrations when working through the percentages section.

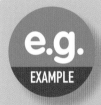

Let me show you an example before having a go yourself:

You have 20 mg of a drug in 8 mL of fluid. What is the concentration in mg/mL? To do this, all we have to do is to divide the drug amount with the volume amount:

$$\frac{20 \text{ mg}}{8 \text{ mL}} = 2.5 \text{ mg/mL}$$

We can reverse check this: 8 lots of 2.5 = 20 (8 × 2.5 = 20)

Activity 2.2

ACTIVITY

1   500 mg Amoxicillin powder is dissolved in 25 mL water for injection. What is the concentration in mg/mL?
2   A syringe contains 20 mg of morphine in 4 mL. What is the concentration in mg/mL?
3   You have 1000 mg of a drug in 20 mL fluid. What is the concentration in mg/mL?

You would have noticed when looking at Question 3 that the names of the drugs did not matter when answering the question as we are looking at the maths aspect only. Sometimes we need to remove the waffle!

DECIMALS

Decimal numbers describe tenths, hundredths and thousandths of a number. For example, 1.25 is equal to one whole unit, plus a fraction of one (25 hundredths). Let me show you this in a visual format:

 Thousands Hundreds Tens Ones Decimal Point Tenths Hundreths Thousanths

| | | | 1 | ● | 2 | 5 |

Whole Numbers   Decimal Fractions

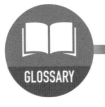

GLOSSARY

Decimal
A decimal is a number that is expressed in the counting system that uses units of tens.

15

Rounding Decimal Numbers

Sometimes it is necessary to 'round up' or 'round down' a decimal number or a whole number. This is particularly true in infusion drip rate calculations, as it is impossible to give a 'point' or part of a drop when setting an infusion rate; for example, 7.2 drops: how would you get the 0.2? Other medication calculations may need to be highly accurate and *incorporate* all the 'points', but as a general rule:

If the number after the point is 4 or less: round down

If the number after the point is 5 or more: round up

This is often known as the 'rule of 5s'.

Therefore, 7.2 drops become 7 drops only; 2.8 becomes 3.

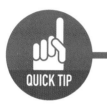

QUICK TIP

I get it! Decimal places are numbers to the right of the decimal point. Example: 5.72 has two decimal places.

Let me show you an example. . .

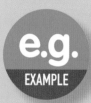

EXAMPLE

39.4 rounds down to **39**

2.82 rounds down to **2.8** (one decimal place)

0.864 rounds down to **0.86** (two decimal places)

31.7 rounds up to **32**

39.8 rounds up to **40**

1.65 rounds up to **1.7** (one decimal place)

0.421 rounds down to **0.42** (two decimal places)

Now, have a go at working some out for yourself: You didn't really expect me to do all the work, did you?

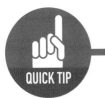

QUICK TIP

Add a zero before the decimal point: for example, .2 should be 0.2, otherwise it could be mistaken for 2.

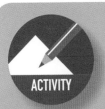

ACTIVITY

Activity 2.3

Round each of the following to one decimal place.

SECTION ONE
1 2.66
2 1.32
3 1.75
4 1.98
5 4.64

Round each of the following to the nearest whole number.

SECTION TWO
1 55.8
2 43.2
3 99.56
4 33.33
5 66.66

NOTE: A cowboy asked me if I could help round up 18 cows. I said 'Yes of course, that's 20 cows.'

PERCENTAGES

Fractions, decimals and percentages all represent parts of a whole. For example:

$$50\% = 0.5 = \frac{1}{2} = \text{one half}$$

A bag of 5% glucose means that there are 5 parts of glucose per 100 parts of water. This can be expressed as a percentage like this: $\dfrac{5}{100}$

'Per cent' means 'per 100'.

Percentage

A percentage is a way of expressing a number as a fraction of 100.

GLOSSARY

Calculating the Percentage of a Number

$$\text{Value} = \frac{\text{number}}{100} \times \text{percentage required}$$

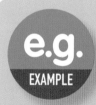

Let me show you an example. . .

e.g.

EXAMPLE

Mrs Noto has to decrease her 160 mL of medication by 15%. How many millilitres has this to be reduced by? In other words, how much of the medication does Mrs Noto now need to take?

Initial Prescription: 160 mL

Dose needs to be decreased by 15%

$$\frac{160}{100} \times 15 = 24 \text{ mL}$$

$$160 \text{ mL minus } 24 \text{ mL} = 136 \text{ mL}$$

Mrs Noto now needs to take 136 mL of the medication.

Finding One Amount as a Percentage of Another

$$\text{Percentage} = \frac{\text{small number}}{\text{larger number}} \times 100$$

NOTE: This is a general rule of thumb, but it should be noted that technically you can get percentages larger than 100%:

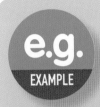

Let me show you an example. . .

EXAMPLE

In a calculations test, 280 student nurses out of 400 passed the test the first time. What percentage was this?

$$\frac{280}{400} \times 100 = 70\%$$

Now have a go at working some examples out for yourself.

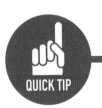

QUICK TIP

Remember: a percentage indicates a number of parts in a hundred.

Activity 2.4

Calculate the following:

1 20% of 450 mL
2 15% of 1200 mL
3 In a numeracy test, 240 out of 300 score more than 50. What percentage is this?
4 In a Clinical Directorate, 85 out of 400 nursing staff are male. What percentage is this?

CONCENTRATIONS

Many medicines come in the form of a solution. A solution contains a solute (the pharmaceutical product) dissolved in a solvent (often liquid). The solution can be dilute or concentrate. An example of this is a strong cider (concentrate) which has now had lemonade added, meaning that the strong cider has been diluted (this drink is called a cider shandy — cheers)!

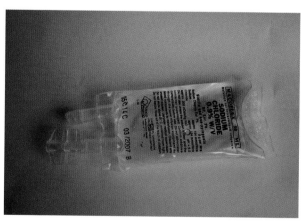

NOTE: did you ever wonder how much 0.9% sodium chloride in grams there is in 1 L of fluid? This is known as weight in volume, or w/v. We work this out:

$$\frac{0.9\%}{100} \times 1000\,mL = 9\,g$$

In a 50 mL bag of fluid, this would equate to 0.45 g (or 450 mg).

$$\frac{0.9\%}{100} \times 50\,mL = 0.45\,g$$

NOTE: In health care we can often see medications expressed as percentage concentrations:

w/w	weight in weight
w/v	weight in volume
v/v	volume in volume

Strength of a Solution

Let me show you examples of these percentage concentration questions:

% weight in weight (w/w)

You have a cream that is 8% Zinc Oxide. How many grams of Zinc Oxide are there in a 30 gram tube of cream?

We work this out in small steps:

Tube size = 30 grams

Percentage amount of medication = 8%

$\frac{30 \times 8}{100}$ = 2.4 grams of Zinc Oxide in 30 grams

% Weight in Volume (w/v)

We need to know how many grams of Dextrose a patient will receive from 2 litres of 5% Dextrose solution.

We can work this out like this:

First, we need to convert 2 litres into mLs = 2000 mLs.

$$\frac{2000 \times 5}{100} = 100 \text{ grams Dextrose}$$

% Volume in Volume (v/v)

To find this percentage we can use the following formula:

$$\frac{\% \text{ solute volume}}{\% \text{ solute volume}} \times 100$$

Let me show you how to use this percentage in practice: A bottle of wine (red, rosé or white – your choice) may have the concentration on the label expressed as v/v%. Wine has about 12 mLs alcohol (ethanol) per 100 mLs of solution. Using our formula above:

$$\frac{12 \text{ mL alcohol}}{100 \text{ mL solution}} \times 100 = 12 \text{ v/v } \% \text{ alcohol.}$$

This is not the end of the story as alcohol is often presented as 'proof'. The proof value is twice the v/v% value, which actually makes the above have a proof value of 24%. Hic!

Some drugs, such as local anesthetics, are also presented in different percentage solutions. To work out how many mg per mL there are in 1% lignocaine, we already know that 1% means 1 in 100.

Convention tells us that 1 mL is equivalent to 1 gram, therefore, 1% lignocaine means that there is 1 g of anesthetic to every 100 mL of the solution.

NOTE: I have never met this person called convention!

This means 1000 mg = 100 mL.

1 mL of 1% lignocaine will therefore contains:

$$\frac{1000}{100} = 10 \, mg \, / \, mL$$

Therefore, 1% of lignocaine is equivalent to 10 mg per mL.

FRACTIONS

Many drug calculations require you to work with fractions. A fraction is a portion of a whole that indicates division into equal parts. For example: one large tablet cut into quarters:

$$\frac{1 \, large \, tablet}{4} = \frac{1}{4}$$

NOTE: when administering medications, tablets should only ever be cut into halves, if the tablet is scored (has a line down its centre). Tablets should *never* be broken into four pieces as this is too inaccurate a dose, as some of the tablet will just crumble away.

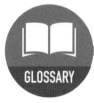

GLOSSARY

Fraction
A fraction represents a part of a whole.

Simplifying Fractions

To cancel down (or simplify) a fraction, you will need to divide the numerator and the denominator by the same number. This is called a common factor.

Example 1:

$$\frac{25}{55} = \frac{5}{11} \text{ Common factor} = 5$$

Example 2:

$$\frac{100}{225} = \frac{4}{9} \text{ Common factor} = 25$$

NOTE:

$$\frac{2}{4} = \frac{3}{6} = \frac{4}{8} = \frac{5}{10}$$

These are all the same as $\frac{1}{2}$, or, expressed another way, 50%.

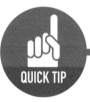

QUICK TIP

The numerator is the top number in a fraction and a denominator is the bottom number.

If you need to add fractions, you can do this in three simple steps. Let me show you an example of adding ¼ to ¼:

1. In this case, the bottom numbers are both 4 (the denominators)

2. Add the top numbers (the numerators) and put this answer on top of the denominators like this:

   1 + 1 = 2, giving us the fraction 2/4

3. We can simplify this fraction if required like this:

   2 goes into 2 once and into 4 twice, leaving us with ½

   Therefore, ¼ added to ¼ equals ½.

Changing Fractions into Decimals

Divide the top number by the bottom number.

Example:

$$\frac{4}{5} = 4 \text{ divided by } 5 = 0.8$$

Activity 2.5

ACTIVITY

Change the following fractions to decimals, giving your answer to one decimal place.

1 $\dfrac{25}{3}$ **2** $\dfrac{15}{2}$ **3** $\dfrac{175}{5}$ **4** $\dfrac{125}{6}$ **5** $\dfrac{250}{6}$ **6** $\dfrac{122}{7}$

Simple Conversions from Fractions, Decimals and Percentages

Let me show you something:

$$\frac{20}{100} \text{ can be broken down to } \frac{2}{10}$$

by removing one zero from the top and one from the bottom.

This can be broken down to '2 goes into 2 once, and 2 goes into 10 five times,' This makes a *simplified fraction*:

$$\frac{1}{5}$$

This is the same as 20%: 20% is one-fifth of 100%, as there are five lots of 20 in 100%.

Fraction	Simplified fraction	How this is expressed in words	Decimals	Percentage
$\frac{10}{100}$	$\frac{1}{10}$	One-tenth	0.1 (0.10)	10%
$\frac{20}{100}$	$\frac{1}{5}$	One-fifth	0.2 (0.20)	20%
$\frac{25}{100}$	$\frac{1}{4}$	One-quarter	0.25	25%
$\frac{33}{100}$	$\frac{1}{3}$	One-third	0.33	33%
$\frac{50}{100}$	$\frac{1}{2}$	One-half	0.5 (0.50)	50%
$\frac{66}{100}$	$\frac{2}{3}$	Two-thirds	0.66	66%
$\frac{75}{100}$	$\frac{3}{4}$	Three-quarters	0.75	75%

RATIOS

A ratio is a way of describing a mixture of two or more components. For example, to mix substances A and B in the ratio 2:1 means that there are two parts of A to every one part of B, making three parts in total: 2 + 1 = 3.

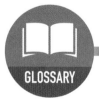

GLOSSARY

Ratio
A ratio is the relative sizes of two or more values.

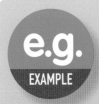

Let me show you an example. . .

A carton of 500 mL of concentrated juice has the instruction 'dilute 7 parts of water to 1 part of juice'. How much juice can be made from this bottle to give to a ward of patients during a heat wave? First, we must pull out the information we need to work this out, and disregard the waffle.

Dilute 7 parts of water to 1 part of juice: this equates to 7:1, which means there are eight parts in total (7 + 1 = 8).

Each part is worth 500 mL.

$$500 \times 1 = 500$$
$$500 \times 7 = 3500$$
$$3500 + 500 = 4000 \, \text{mL in total.}$$

or

$$500 \, \text{mL} \times 8 = 4000 \, \text{mL} \, (\text{or} \, 4 \, \text{L})$$

A strength of a solution may also be given as a ratio as 1 *in* 4. This means that 1 part of stock solution has been added in 3 parts of diluted solution.

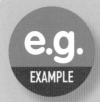

Let me show you an example. . .

The ratio 1 in 10 means that there is one part stock solution to every nine parts of dilutant: 10 parts in total. 10 minus 1 = 9 parts of dilutant, therefore 1 in 10 equates to 1:9.

Therefore, 1 in 4 means 1 part of stock solution added in 4 parts of diluted solution.

1:3 means one part of stock solution added to three parts of dilutant.

Don't worry, let's look at another one: a learning disabilities nurse is taking her client to a swimming session. The pool is 20 m wide and 50 m long. What is the simplest ratio of the pool's width to its length?

Both the 20 and the 50 can be divided by 10:

$$20 / 10 = 2$$
$$50 / 10 = 5$$

Therefore, the simplest form of the ratio is **2:5**.

NOTE: Adrenaline for anaphylaxis is expressed as 1:1000. This means that there is 1 mg for every 1 mL (1 mg/mL), which is equivalent to *1 g in every 1000 mL*. Therefore, if we were to administer 0.5 mg of the drug, we would need to give 0.5 mL.

Adrenaline for cardiac arrest is expressed as 1:10 000. This means that there is 1 mg in 10 mL (or 0.1 mg for every 1 mL), or *1 g in 10 000 mL*. As we administer the whole 10 mL of the drug, we are giving 10 times the volume than for anaphylaxis situations (10 mL).

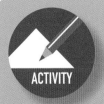

Activity 2.6

ACTIVITY

You have two solutions of Adrenaline: 1 in 1000 and 1 in 10 000
1   What is the concentration of both strengths in mg/mL?
2   Which solution is the weakest?

See how you get on in Activity 2.7. Don't go peeking at the answers: have a go first!

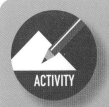

Activity 2.7

1 How much stock solution is present in 100 mL of diluted solution if expressing this as the ratio (i) 1 in 4 and (ii) 1:4?

2 How much stock solution is present in 5 L of diluted solution if expressing this as the ratio (i) 1 in 9 and (ii) 1:9?

3 How much stock solution is present in 550 mL of diluted solution if expressing this as the ratio (i) 1 in 10 and (ii) 1:10?

4 How much stock solution is present in 600 mL of diluted solution if expressing this as the ratio (i) 1 in 3 and (ii) 1:3?

AVERAGES

An average may be a mode, median, range or mean:

- **mode:** the most common figure in a series of figures;
- **median:** the figure in the centre of a series of values placed in order;
- **range:** the lowest to the highest value;
- **mean:** most commonly referred to as the 'average'. All values added together and divided by the number of units.

Let me show you an example. . .

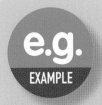

Brendan Topa's temperature during the day has been:

06:00	37.2°C (degrees Celsius)		
08:00	37.2°C	16:00	38.0°C
10:00	37.8°C	18:00	37.6°C
12:00	38.0°C	20:00	37.4°C
14:00	38.0°C	22:00	37.0°C

What is the mode?

38.0°C, as there are three recordings of this figure.

What is the median?

37.0	37.2	37.2	37.4	37.6
37.8	38.0	38.0	38.0	

The median is 37.6 when the values are placed in numerical order.

What is the range?

37.0–38.0: the smallest figure to the largest figure is the difference of one whole degree celsius (1°C).

What is the mean?

$$37.2 + 37.2 + 37.8 + 38.0 + 38.0 + 38.0 + 37.6 + 37.4 + 37.0 =$$
$$3382 / 9 \left(\text{number of units}\right) = 37.57777 = 37.6°C$$

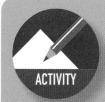

Activity 2.8

ACTIVITY

1   What is the mean average of Judith Goodman's intracranial pressure recordings? **NOTE**: intracranial pressure is the pressure of cerebrospinal fluid within the ventricles and subarachnoid space in the brain (I know, too much information!).

08:00	19 mmHg
09:00	19 mmHg
10:00	19.5 mmHg
11:00	18.0 mmHg
12:00	17 mmHg

KEY POINTS

- Revising calculation basics in adding, subtracting, dividing and multiplying.
- Revising calculation basics in decimals, converting units, percentages, fractions, ratios and averages.
- Looking at different ways a strength of a solution can be expressed.

USEFUL WEB RESOURCES

http://www.bbc.co.uk/schools/gcsebitesize/maths/number/
http://www.mathsisfun.com

Chapter 3
. . . .
METRIC UNITS AND CONVERSIONS

Calculation Skills for Nurses, Second Edition. Claire Boyd.
© 2022 John Wiley & Sons Ltd. Published 2022 by John Wiley & Sons Ltd.

METRIC MEASURES

The metric system is based on multiples of 10. We will look at metric units of length later on in this chapter but first we will look at **metric measures of weight.**

So, for weight:

1 kilogram (kg)	= 1000 grams (g)
1 gram (g)	= 1000 milligrams (mg)
1 milligram (mg)	= 1000 micrograms
1 microgram	= 1000 nanograms (ng)
1 nanogram (ng)	= 1000 picograms (pg)

NOTE: where medications are concerned micrograms should *not* be abbreviated on prescription charts to mcg. This is due to the abbreviations for milligram (mg) and microgram (mcg) being quite similar, and they may be misread by the person administering the drug. As a nurse you may also see **µ**, which is another way of writing 'micro'. So, **µ**g means micrograms.

Nanograms and picograms are very small units indeed (and are very rarely used in prescriptions).

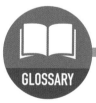

GLOSSARY

Nanogram
A nanogram is equal to one billionth of a gram = 0. 000 000 001 grams.

Metric Weights
Metric weights are a decimal unit of weight based on the gram.

Conversion from One Unit to Another

In drug calculations it is best to work in whole numbers – that is, 125 micrograms and not 0.125 mg – as fewer mistakes may be made. Therefore. it is necessary to be able to convert easily from one unit to another. To do this you have to multiply or divide by a thousand.

Converting Larger Units to the Next Smaller Unit

To convert a LARGER unit to a smaller unit you multiply by 1000.

NOTE: the × symbol means multiply.

To multiply by 1000, you may wish to just move the decimal point three places to the right.

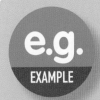

Let me show you an example. . .

Convert 5 g to milligrams: 5 × 1000 = 5000 mg

Convert 0.25 kg to grams: 0.25 × 1000 = 250 g

This can be done another way, simply by 'bouncing' the decimal point.

To multiply by 1000, you move the decimal point three places to the right.

Changing 5 g to milligrams: 5 .0 0 0 g = 5000 mg

Converting Smaller Units to the Next Larger Unit

To convert a SMALLER unit to the next larger unit you divide by 1000.

NOTE: the / symbol = Divided by.

To divide by 1000, you may just wish to move the decimal point three places to the left.

Let me show you an example. . .

EXAMPLE

Convert 6000 g to kilograms: 6000/1000 = 6 kg

Convert 325 mg to grams: 325/1000 = 0.325 g

To bounce using the decimal point method.

To divide by 1000, you move the decimal point three places to the left.

Changing 5000 mg to grams: 5000.0 mg = 5 g

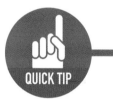

QUICK TIP

Once you have written a decimal point in your result, any noughts at the end of the answer become unnecessary.

For example: 0.6000 is written as 0.6.

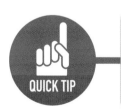

QUICK TIP

Here is a quick way of remembering this: going up to larger units: divide and move decimal place to the left ↑ ÷ ←·

going down to smaller units: multiply and move decimal place to the right ↓ × · →

For volume, we need to know that:

$$1\,\text{litre}\,(\text{L}) = 1000\,\text{millilitres}\,(\text{mL})$$

Now let's have a go at converting some metric units:

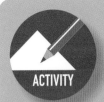

Activity 3.1

SECTION ONE

1 6000 mg to grams
2 39 000 mL to litres
3 350 mL to litres
4 0.07 micrograms to milligrams
5 4000 g to kilograms
6 4500 mg to grams
7 0.8 mg to micrograms
8 9 micrograms to nanograms
9 1300 g to kilograms
10 0.462 mg to grams

SECTION TWO

1 0.72 g to mg
2 1.4 mg to micrograms
3 0.03 g to milligrams
4 2 g to kilograms
5 2.5 L to millilitres
6 0.7 mg to micrograms
7 61.25 L to millilitres
8 92 kg to grams
9 0.02 mg to micrograms
10 0.023 mg to grams

SECTION THREE

1 20 micrograms to mg
2 634 g to kilograms
3 0.0635 mg to micrograms
4 0.25 micrograms to nanograms
5 8 kg to grams
6 1527 micrograms to milligrams
7 21.9 L to millilitres
8 64.5 micrograms to milligrams
9 349.8 g to kilograms
10 50 mL to litres

SECTION FOUR

1 3 L to millilitres
2 1.2 mg to micrograms
3 0.04 mg to micrograms
4 0.12 g to milligrams
5 0.02 mg to grams
6 0.02 micrograms to nanograms
7 2.386 kg to grams
8 4 ng to micrograms
9 1234 mL to litres
10 320 mg to grams

It may be necessary to convert imperial weights into metric weights, i.e., stones and pounds into kilograms, or vice versa. We need to know that:

$$1\,pound = 0.45\,kg$$
$$1\,stone = 6.35\,kg, and$$
$$1\,kg = 2.2\,pounds\,(lb)$$

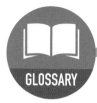

Imperial Weights

Imperial weights are a system of units using stones, pounds and ounces.

GLOSSARY

For example, a patient weighs 9 stone, 5 lb. To convert this to the metric system, you could take the 9 stone and multiply this by 6.35 kg = 57.15 kg. Then take the 5 lb and multiply this by 0.45 kg = 2.25 kg. Add these together (57.15 + 2.25 kg). Therefore, 9 stone, 5 lb = 59.40 kg. Just to note, you could just look at the conversion table in Appendix 5 – but where would the fun be in not working this out yourself?

Are you ready for some more exercises? Who said no?

Activity 3.2

ACTIVITY

1 Change 3000 mg to grams.
2 Change 38 000 mL to litres.
3 Change 250 mL to litres.
4 Change 0.05 micrograms to milligrams.
5 Change 2000 g to kilograms.
6 Change 2500 mg to grams.
7 Change 0.3 mg to micrograms.
8 Change 6 micrograms to nanograms.
9 Change 1600 g to kilograms.
10 Change 0.375 mg to grams.
11 A patient weighs 15 stone, 10 lb. What is this in kilograms?
12 A patient weighs 82.55 kg and asks you what this is 'in old money', meaning in stones?
13 A patient has taken two doses of her 400 microgram glyceryl trinitrate spray. How many milligrams has she taken?

14 Change 0.075 mg to micrograms.

15 Change 935 grams to kilograms.

16 Digoxin tablets are presented as 125 micrograms. What is this in milligrams?

17 Change 1.4 litres to millilitres.

18 Change 27 mg to grams.

19 A patient has taken 0.75 g of medication. How much is this in milligrams?

20 Change 7 ng into picograms.

Picogram

A picogram is equal to one trillionth of a gram.

METRIC UNITS OF LENGTH

Units of length most often used by nurses are metres and centimetres. Just like units of weight, such as kilograms/ grams, etc, you may need to convert a larger unit into a smaller unit, i.e., metres into centimetres. It is important to know how to do this correctly as collecting a patient's height and weight can be used to assess their Body Mass Index (BMI), which you can learn more about on Chapter 13. Height and weight are also used on paediatric units for baby's growth charts, known as centile charts.

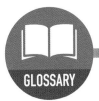

Centile Charts

A centile chart tracks baby's physical development by measuring weight, length and head circumference and plotting this on the chart.

Once when I asked my group of students what we need to do to change centimetres into metres, I was told to 'just remove the "centi" and voila – metres' – not quite what I was looking for, but good attempt!

> **REMEMBER:**
> 1 metre = 100 cm.
> 1 metre = 1000 mm
> 1 cm = 10 mm
> For this reason, you need to:

Convert larger metres (m) into smaller centimetres (cm), you need to multiply the metre figure by 100 = cm.

Convert larger metres (m) into even smaller millimetres (mm), you need to multiply the metre figure by 1000 = mm.

Convert small centimetres (cm) into even smaller millimetres (mm), you need to multiply the centimetre figure by 10 = mm.

For visual learners; when needing to go down metric units:

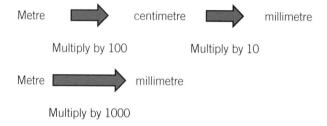

Metre ⟹ centimetre ⟹ millimetre

Multiply by 100   Multiply by 10

Metre ⟹ millimetre

Multiply by 1000

When needing to go up metric units we are going the other way and instead of multiplying we divide – this is all the same principle as when converting metric weights at the start of this chapter.

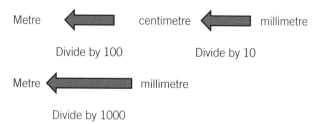

Metre ⟸ centimetre ⟸ millimetre

Divide by 100   Divide by 10

Metre ⟸ millimetre

Divide by 1000

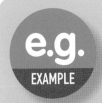

Let me show you some length conversion examples:

EXAMPLE

1 Convert baby Owen's height measurement from 1.15 m into centimetres.

ANSWER: As we are going DOWN from metres to the next metric unit we need to multiply by 100.

$1.15 \text{ m} \times 100 = 115 \text{ cm.}$

2 Convert baby Rhys height measurement from 0.98 m into centimetres.

ANSWER: As we are going DOWN from metres to the next metric unit we need to multiply by 100.

$0.98 \text{ m} \times 100 = 98 \text{ cm.}$

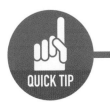

QUICK TIP

Did you remember that you can use the decimal point bounce method from the beginning of this chapter?

ACTIVITY

Activity 3.3

Convert these patients' heights into centimetres:

1 Patient 1 is 975 mm
2 Patient 2 is 1.27 m
3 Patient 3 is 325 mm
4 Patient 4 is 1.08 m
5 Patient 5 is 617 mm

Convert these patients' heights into millimetres:

6 Patient 6 is 1.13 m
7 Patient 7 is 1.02 m
8 Patient 8 is 0.77 m
9 Patient 9 is 0.981 m
10 Patient 10 is 1.90 m

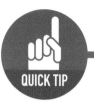

QUICK TIP

Don't forget to ask yourself, does my answer look right?

KEY POINTS

- Looking at metric and imperial weights.
- Looking at how to convert metric units and volumes.
- Looking at metric units of length

USEFUL WEB RESOURCES

http://www.bbc.co.uk/schools/gcsebitesize/maths/number
http://www.mathsisfun.com/measure/metric-syste.html

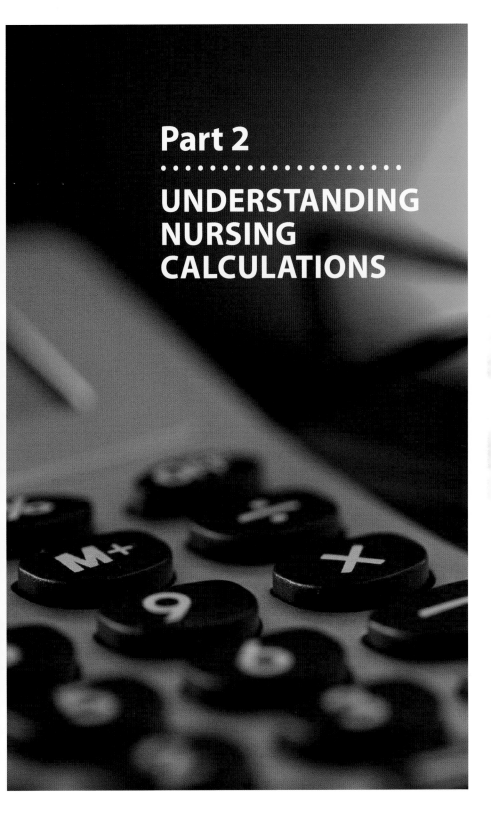

Part 2
UNDERSTANDING NURSING CALCULATIONS

Chapter 4

· · · · · · · · · · · · · · · · · · · ·

TABLETS
AND CAPSULES

Calculation Skills for Nurses, Second Edition. Claire Boyd.
© 2022 John Wiley & Sons Ltd. Published 2022 by John Wiley & Sons Ltd.

LEARNING OUTCOMES

By the end of this chapter you should be familiar with the formula 'what you want divided by what you have' (or similar wording) and calculating the total amount of tablets or capsules you require from a prescription.

When working out how many tablets or capsules to administer for drug administration, some calculations can be quite simple:

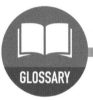

GLOSSARY

Capsule

A capsule is a soluble container enclosing a dose of medicine.

Paracetamol is presented as 500 mg per tablet.

If a patient requires (is prescribed) 1000 mg we can see that two tablets are required (500 mg + 500 mg = 1000 mg). This is known as the calculations 'bundles' approach.

Or, we can use a formula:

$$\text{Number of tables or capsules required} = \frac{\text{what you want}}{\text{what you've got}}$$

This means what you want divided by what you've got.

The formula approach comes into its own when we have more complicated calculations to work out. However, an understanding of the whys and wherefores of the problem must first be established: that is, what are we doing and why? We should always also be thinking around the box: does the answer look right? This means we should already have made a rough estimate (or 'guesstimation') of the answer.

NOTE: 'what you want' is what has been prescribed and we divide this by how the medication is presented in its blister pack or bottle, which is the 'what you've got' part.

It is important to use the wording that makes sense to you. Some people prefer to use these different expressions:

- What you need divided by what it comes in.
- Dose prescribed divided by dose you have available.
- Strength required divided by stock strength.
- What you desire divided by what is at hand.
- Amount desired divided by amount you have.

NOTE: it is important that w we are using a formula all the metric units are the same. For example, if 'what you want' is in milligrams then the 'what you've got' has also got to be in milligrams. Now it should make sense why we have spent so much time on conversions in the previous chapters!

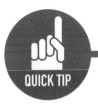

I think the wording I'll use is 'prescription divided by amount per tablet/capsule'. This makes sense to me.

Let me show you an example. . .

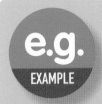

You pick up the prescription chart and see that a patient has been prescribed 225 mg of a drug. This is the **what you want** part of the formula.

Two tablets of the prescribed drug are in a blister pack in the stock cupboard. This is **what you've got** part of the formula. Each tablet is equal to 150 mg of the drug. Visualise yourself getting the drug out of the cupboard and popping the pills into a medicine pot. But you know two of these tablets will be too much, i.e., more than what the prescription asked for.

So, you put the figures into the formula and, if using a calculator, input: 225 mg (what you want) divided by 150 mg (what you've got) = 1.5 = 1½ tablets. Therefore, one of the tablets needs to be split in half. Simples!

NOTE: remember what we said about cutting tablets in half: do so only if they are scored, and never cut a tablet into quarters.

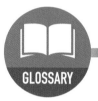

Prescription Chart

A prescription chart is a legal document under the UK Medicines Act 1968. It is a written direction of prescribed drugs.

GLOSSARY

Now have a go at working through some of these yourself, using the formula given above.

ACTIVITY

Activity 4.1a

In each case, calculate how many tablets or capsules are required.

1   Prescribed: 60 mg codeine phosphate; stock strength: 30 mg
2   Prescribed: 75 mg aspirin; stock strength: 150 mg aspirin
3   Prescribed: 225 mg ranitidine; stock strength: 150 mg
4   Prescribed: 0.5 micrograms daily (very small dose); stock strength: 250 mg (quite large dose). Is this really achievable? Remember, medics can make mistakes when writing prescriptions. Trust yourself.
5   What you want: 5 mg timolol maleate; what you've got: 10 mg
6   What you need: 15 mg nortriptyline; how it comes: 10 mg

Number of tablets: tablets may be available in different strengths and you should always give as few as possible, in the best combination (who likes swallowing pills at the best of times?).

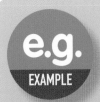

Let me show you an example. . .

Tablets are presented as 10 mg, 5 mg, 2 mg and 1 mg. Working out the best combination for the following prescriptions show that:

1   Patient prescribed 11 mg = 10 mg + 1 mg = 2 tablets
2   Patient prescribed 8 mg = 5 mg + 2 mg + 1 mg = 3 tablets
3   Patient prescribed 12 mg = 10 mg + 2 mg = 2 tablets
4   Patient prescribed 4 mg = 2 mg + 2 mg = 2 tablets

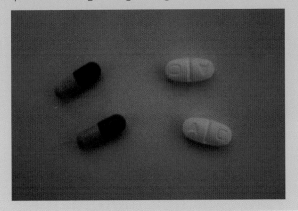

Want some more questions to practice on? Go on, you know you want to!

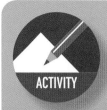

Activity 4.1b

1   Patient has been prescribed 125 micrograms of digoxin. You have 62.5 microgram tablets in stock. How many tablets do you give?

2   Warfarin tablets, in stock, are presented as 0.5 mg, 1 mg, 2 mg and 5 mg. Your patient is prescribed 9 mg. Which tablets do you administer for the required prescription?

3   Prescribed: 300 mg cimetidine. What you've got: 200 mg. How many tablets do you give?

4   Verapamil tablets come in strengths of 40 mg, 80 mg, 120 mg and 160 mg. A patient is prescribed 320 mg of the drug. Which tablets do you administer for the required prescription?

5   Prescribed: 75 mg thioridazine. You have 10 mg, 25 mg, 50 mg and 100 mg strengths in stock. Which tablets do you administer for the required prescription?

6   A patient has been prescribed 250 mg of chlorpropamide, to be administered with breakfast. Presently on the ward there are only 100 mg tablets obtainable. How many tablets do you give?

TOTAL DAILY DOSES

Sometimes a drug is written as a Total Daily Dose (TDD) in a patient's medical notes. The prescriber may then need to divide this up into two, three or four equal doses, if a single dose is too large to take in one go. It is important to check a prescription to establish whether a prescription is a TDD or a single dose we should be administering. This is where we will see the Latin abbreviations bd, tds or qds – please look at page xiii at the front of the book, but generally:

- Bd means a medicine is to be administered twice a day, e.g., 10 am and 10 pm
- Tds means a medicine is to be administered three times a day, e.g., 8 am, 4 pm and 12 mid-night
- Qds means a medicine is to be administered four times a day, e.g., 6 am, 12 mid-day, 6 pm and 12 mid-night

Sometimes the TDD is worked out according to the patient's body weight in kg (what we call titrated), which we will look at in Chapter 8, but let me show you an example now:

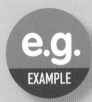

A patient has been prescribed Amoxicillin 55 mg /kg/day. The patient weighs 50 kg. How many mg of the Amoxicillin will you give the patient for the whole day?

ANSWER: This is where I multiply the patient's weight in kgs by the drug dose:

Dose × Weight (kg)

55 mg × 50 kg = 2750

Therefore. the TDD is 2750 mg

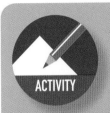

Activity 4.2

A patient has been prescribed Chloramphenicol 25 mg/kg/day in 4 divided doses. The patient weighs 65 kg.
(1) What is her Total Daily Dose (TDD)?
(2) What is the single dose?

Remember:

(a) is a simple multiplication

(b) is a simple division

KEY POINTS

- Looking at the formula used to work out how many tablets or capsules to administer according to the prescribed prescription.
- Working out how to administer the smallest number of tablets or capsules for the dose prescribed.
- Looking at Total Daily Doses

USEFUL WEB RESOURCES

http://www.bbc.co.uk/schools/gcsebitesize/maths/number/
http://www.bnf.org/bnf/bnf/current/104945.htm
You will need to register to access the bnf site (but registration is free)

Chapter 5

. . . .

LIQUIDS AND INJECTABLES

Calculation Skills for Nurses, Second Edition. Claire Boyd.
© 2022 John Wiley & Sons Ltd. Published 2022 by John Wiley & Sons Ltd.

LEARNING OUTCOMES

By the end of this chapter you should be familiar with the formula 'what you want divided by what you've got multiplied by the volume' (or similar wording) and be able to calculate the amount of drug (in millilitres) you require from a prescription. You will also have an understanding of the ratio approach to work this out. You will also have a working knowledge of how to use a calculator.

All injections (subcutaneous, intramuscular, intravenous, etc.) need to be in a liquid form (as it's difficult to push a dry tablet into someone's veins or muscle!).

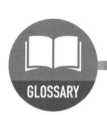
GLOSSARY

Intradermal Injection
Liquid medication administered between the layers of the skin.

Subcutaneous Injection
Liquid medication administered into the fatty tissue directly below the skin.

Intramuscular Injection
Liquid medication inserted into the central area of a specific muscle.

Intravenous Injection
Liquid medication administered through an access device directly into a vein.

So, these medications have been mixed in a transport medium (the liquid). Volume = liquid.

Let's imagine we have a 2 mg tablet. It is to be injected into the patient's muscle, so we use a mortar and pestle and crush the drug and then add the transport medium, water.

NOTE: we would not do this in practice! If we add 1 ml of water, the drug is said to be presented as 2 mg/1 mL. If we add 10 mL of water, then the drug is said to be 2 mg/10 mL. If we add 1000 mL (or 1 L) to the crushed tablet, the drug is said to be 2 mg/1 L. The important thing to note is that the drug amount has not changed, only the volume. Don't lose sight of the fact that in the last case we would still have a 2 mg tablet floating around in 1 L of liquid.

To work out how many mg of a drug is in 1mL of the fluid, we can use the ratio approach.

Here is an example of the ratio approach:

Sodium Valporate solution contains 200 mg in 5 mL. Using the ratio approach we can work out that there is 40 mg in every 1 mL (200 mg/5 mL = 40 mg) and we can build this up on paper to 10 mL:

40 mg = 1 mL

80 mg = 2 mL

120 mg = 3mL

160 mg = 4 mL

200 mg = 5 mL

240mg = 6 mL

280 mg = 7 mL

320 mg = 8 mL

360 mg = 9 mL

400 mg = 10 mL

So, if a patient is prescribed 400 mg per dose, we can see that we need to draw up 10 mL for the prescription.

I prefer the formula approach of What you Want, divided by What you're Got multiplied by the Volume:

$$\frac{WYW}{WYG} \times Vol \quad \frac{400 \text{ mg}}{200 \text{ mg}} \times 5mL = 10 \text{ mL}$$

As you can see, we can use the same formula as we used for dry dosages (see Chapter 4), but we now need to add the volume part to it:

$$\frac{\text{Volume of drug}}{\text{to be given}} = \frac{\text{what you want}}{\text{what you've got}} \times \text{volume}$$

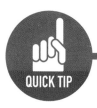

The answer will always be in millilitres now, as the drug is in a liquid form.

NOTE: this formula also works with other liquids, so it does not just apply to injectables, for example, cough syrups, elixirs and linctus.

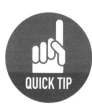

Perhaps you would like to use the formula:
NHS (National Health Service)
N
H × S
N = Need
H = Have
S = Solution

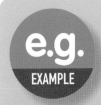

Let me show you an example. . .

A patient has been prescribed 8 mg of morphine and stock ampoules contain 10 mg/mL. What I want = 8 mg, what I've got = 10 mg and what it comes in (volume) = 1 mL:

8 mg divided by 10 mg multiplied by 1 mL = 0.8 mL

So, I draw up 0.8 mL knowing that there is 8 mg of the drug in my syringe.

Looking at the whole picture, I know this looks about right as my answer should indeed be *under* the 1 mL mark, as this is how much liquid holds 10 mg of the drug, and I want less than this.

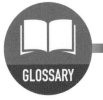

Ampoule
An ampoule is a sealed glass or plastic bulb containing a solution for hypodermic injection.

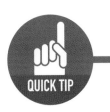

Liquid preparations are very common in baby and infant care.

Activity 5.1

1. Gentamicin is dispensed as 80 mg in 2 mL. The prescription is to administer 50 mg of gentamicin. What volume of gentamicin do you administer?
2. Intravenous (or IV) metronidazole 500 mg is dispensed in a 100 ml bag. A 12-year-old child is prescribed 400 mg of metronidazole. What volume do you administer?
3. Heparin is dispensed as 25 000 units in 1 mL. 20 000 units of heparin is prescribed. What volume do you administer? (There is more about heparin, and units, in Chapter 6.)
4. Teicoplanin comes as 400 mg in 3 mL. A patient is prescribed 600 mg. How many millilitres do you give?
5. A patient is having an anaphylaxis episode (a severe allergic reaction) and requires adrenaline urgently. Adrenaline is presented as 1 mg in 1 mL (1:1000). You are required to administer 500 micrograms intramuscularly (or IM) now, and another 500 micrograms in 5 minutes' time. How much adrenaline (in milligrams and millilitres) do you administer in total?
6. Fluoxetine is presented as 20 mg/5 mL. A patient has been prescribed 30 mg. What volume do you administer?
7. Benzylpenicillin is presented in stock ampoules of 1.2 g in 6 mL of solution. A patient is prescribed 800 mg. What volume do you administer?

In the following, what volume of drug do you administer?

8. Prescribed: 250 mg oral suspension of amoxicillin; stock strength: 125 mg in 5 mL
9. Prescribed: atropine 0.5 mg; stock strength: 0.6 mg/mL
10. Prescribed: 1750 units of heparin; stock strength: 1000 units per mL

Some drugs have to be injected over a given time period, so as not to cause 'speed shock'. For example, furosemide should not exceed 4 mg of the drug over 1 minute.

Speed shock
Speed shock is a sudden, adverse physiological reaction to IV medication administered too quickly.

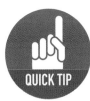

QUICK TIP

Speed shock can be caused by even very small amounts of a drug.

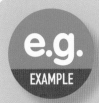

e.g.

EXAMPLE

Let me show you an example. . .

20 mg of furosemide is prescribed and drawn up, but the rate of administration should be no more than 4 mg of the drug over 1 minute, according to British National Formulary (BNF) instructions. This is the formula you may wish to use:

$$\text{Time needed to administer drug} = \frac{\text{dose prescribed}}{\text{rate}}$$

$$\frac{20\text{ mg}}{4\text{ mg}} = 5\text{ min}$$

We will need to inject the furosemide over 5 minutes.

If using a calculator to make this calculation, you take the amount prescribed and divide it by the rate: 20 mg divided by 4 mg = 5. The answer will be in minutes, as this is the formula for giving us times (in minutes).

CALCULATORS

If you wish to use a calculator, get used to inputting numbers into it and remember that some calculators are 'scientific', and so will have lots of buttons that you may not recognise. Some simple calculators do not have a square root button, but in case if you ever need to work out body surface areas it is a good idea to get a calculator with such a button. It looks like this:

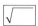

Whatever calculator you use, you will need to get used to using this tool, as many errors occur during the inputting stage. Always read the manufacturer's instructions after purchasing your calculator and practise using it with some sample questions to which you already know the answer before using it in real life. Remember, always ask yourself whether the answer looks right, and get it checked.

Let me show you an example. . .

EXAMPLE

To find 20% of 75, input:

| 2 | 0 | × | 7 | 5 | % | = | 15 |

Therefore, 20% of 75 is 15. Did you notice that you did not need to press the equals (=) button (this may have lead to a wrong answer). To check our answer, we can reverse our findings:

15	=	20%
15	=	20%
15	=	20%
15	=	20%
15	=	20%
		100%

Five bundles of 15 make our 75, which makes up our 100%, so 15 is correct.

NOTE: if your calculator does not have a percentage button, then you just input: 20/100 × 75 = 15.

KEY POINTS

- Looking at the formula used to work out the amount of millilitres to administer volumes according to the prescribed prescription.
- Looking at the ratio approach to work out the amount of millilitres to administer volumes according to the prescribed prescription.
- Becoming conversant with the different types of injection.
- Understanding the basic principles of speed shock in relation to administering IV medications.
- How to input data into a calculator.

USEFUL WEB RESOURCES

http://www.bbc.co.uk/schools/gcsebitesize/maths/number/
http://www.bnf.org/bnf/bnf/current/104945.htm

You will need to register to access the bnf site (but registration is free)

Chapter 6
· ·
SYRINGES AND MENISCUS

Calculation Skills for Nurses, Second Edition. Claire Boyd.
© 2022 John Wiley & Sons Ltd. Published 2022 by John Wiley & Sons Ltd.

LEARNING OUTCOMES

By the end of this chapter you will be aware of the calibrations attributed to the various-sized syringes and syringe types. You will also have an understanding of injection needles and the meniscus effect.

When looking at nursing calculations, it is important that we know how to read the calibrations on syringes. After all, if we have worked out correctly how much of a drug to draw up, we need to then draw up the right amount of drug into our syringe.

Syringes are used to inject medications via the intradermal (within the skin), subcutaneous, intramuscular or intravenous routes. In the neurosciences, medics also use a route known as intrathecal, or within the meninges of the spinal cord. There are many reasons why we would need to give patients their medication with a syringe and needle using one of these routes. For example, patients may be unable to swallow and or unable to tolerate medications and fluid via the oral enteral route, or the prescribed medication may not come in an oral formulation (such as insulin), being destroyed by chemicals in the intestine. An injection of analgesia is more quickly absorbed by the body than a tablet or capsule, which is again the rationale for an injectable format to be chosen. Not all syringes will need to have a needle attached when administering a drug, as we do have oral syringes, often used in paediatrics to measure and administer oral medications. *Oral syringes are not the same as other syringes.*

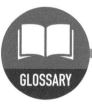

GLOSSARY

Enteral route
The enteral route refers to the administration of a drug directly into the stomach and intestines.

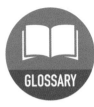

GLOSSARY

Analgesia
Analgesia is medication that reduces or eliminates pain.

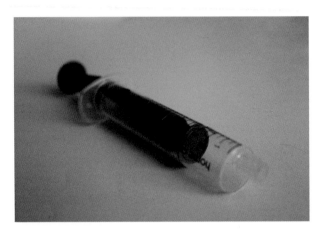

An oral syringe.

THE SYRINGE

The syringe consists of a barrel to contain the liquid that is drawn up, with calibrations marked along the outer surface.

The moveable plunger is contained inside the barrel and has an end tip. Pulling this plunger back sucks fluid into the barrel and pushing this in, or forward, expels the fluid.

The syringe has an end tip, or different varieties and placement, in order for a needle to be attached.

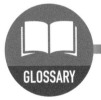

GLOSSARY

Calibration
Calibration refers to marks with a standard scale of readings.

Types of Syringe

Luer-lock   This is used for secure connections, whereby the needle is screwed onto the syringe.

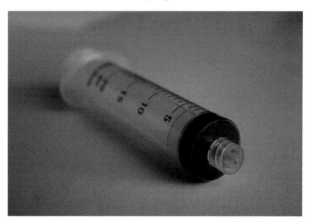

A Luer-lock syringe.

Eccentric Luer-slip   This is where the nozzle is off-centre to allow closer application to the skin.

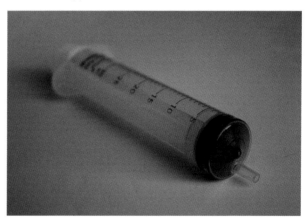

An eccentric Luer-slip syringe.

Concentric Luer-slip   This is used for all other applications. The nozzle is in the centre.

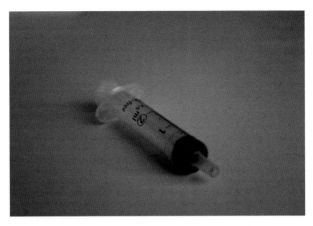

A concentric Luer-slip syringe.

Syringes come in various sizes with different calibrations:

> 1 mL syringes have divisions of 0.01 mL
>
> 2 mL syringes have divisions of 0.1 mL
>
> 5 mL syringes have divisions of 0.2 mL
>
> 10 mL, 20 mL and 50 mL syringes have 1 mL divisions

Insulin

Insulin syringes are used to administer insulin, which is prepared as units per millilitre, in vials that contain 100 units/mL: these are known as multi-dose vials. The standard insulin syringe is calibrated in 2-unit divisions up to 100 units. Patients may require only a small dose (less than 50 units) and so there are also low-dose syringes available which are graduated in 1-unit divisions up to 50 units (in 0.5 mL syringes).

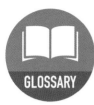

Insulin

Insulin is a hormone that lowers the level of glucose in the blood.

Heparin

Like insulin, heparin is prescribed in units and drawn up in 1 mL syringes, or comes in pre-filled syringes. Heparin is available in single or multi-dose vials, in variable strengths, such as:

1000 units/mL

5000 units/mL

25 000 units/mL

5000 units/5 mL

25 000 units/5 mL

Heparin

Heparin is an anticoagulant medication (anti-blood clotting).

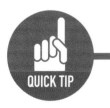

You may still see some medics writing units on prescription charts as IU, meaning International Units. This can be confused with IV for intravenous, so the word units is now preferred.

Don't confuse units with millilitres!

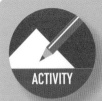

Activity 6.1

1   Mark 30.0 mL on this 50 mL syringe.

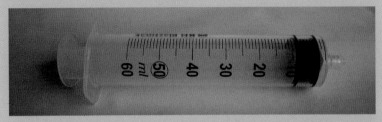

2   Mark 0.75 mL on this syringe.

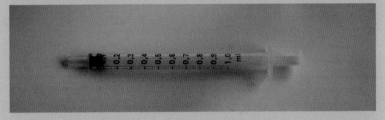

3   How much has been drawn up in this syringe?

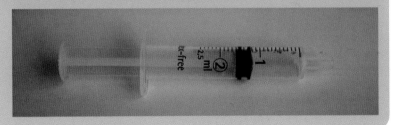

NOTE: a syringe should ideally only be filled to 75% capacity. This is in order for any re-adjustments to be made when drawing up, and is especially true when injecting into muscle, and drawing back to establish that we are not about to inject the medication into a blood vessel. You may have noticed that the 50 mL syringe goes up to 60 mL graduations.

When drawing up medication from an ampoule or vial, ideally a specialised blunt filter needle should be used, but these may not be readily available. Therefore, it is considered best practice to use a quite small needle, to reduce the effect of drawing up shards of glass or particles of the rubber from these receptacles. After the medication has been drawn up, the needle should be replaced with the appropriate-sized needle prior to administration.

Needle Gauge Sizes

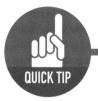

QUICK TIP

The larger the number on a needle, the smaller the needle.

The three most common needles you may use in practice are:

40 mm (21 gauge, or g) = quite large needle

25 mm (23 g) = quite small needle

16 mm (25 g) = very small needle, often used for
subcutaneous injections

The higher the gauge, the finer the bore.

INJECTIONS

The routes most commonly used for the administration of injections are the subcutaneous (SC; beneath the skin), the intramuscular (IM; into muscle) and the intravenous (IV; into a vein) routes. The buttocks tend to be the most common site for IM injections, but due to the presence of nerves in this region, especially the sciatic nerve, this may give rise to nerve damage. The sites used for IM injections tend to be the deltoid (arm), ventrogluteal, dorsogluteal (both buttock muscles, the upper outer quadrant of the buttock) and vastus lateralis (middle outer aspect of the thigh) muscles. Study these muscles in a book on anatomy and physiology.

Subcutaneous injections are administered into the subcutaneous tissue rather than a muscle. Medications administered into this tissue have a slow and steady absorption and blood vessels and nerves are minimal in these areas. The sites most commonly used for subcutaneous injections are the middle outer aspect of the upper arm, the middle anterior aspect of the thigh or the anterior abdominal wall just below the umbilicus.

Needles for Injection

Needles consist of a hub and the tip of the needle is bevelled: this is a 'cut out'. The bevel is uppermost when injecting for intradermal injections, and downwards for all other injections. IM injections into the buttocks tend to be with either a 21 g or 23 g needle. The size of needle depends on the patient's size: 21 g is suitable for most adults and obese adults, whereas 23 g is suitable for very thin adults.

For IM injections into the thigh and arm, the 23 g is suitable for most adults.

For SC injections, the 25 g tends to be used.

Meniscus

Surface tension of a liquid causes it to produce a curved surface as the liquid climbs up the sides of a container. This is called the meniscus. To accurately measure the liquid in a medicine pot or syringe you read the bottom of the curve of the meniscus, where it is at its lowest, in the middle (the bottom of the meniscus), not the top of the curve (top of the meniscus).

Activity 6.2

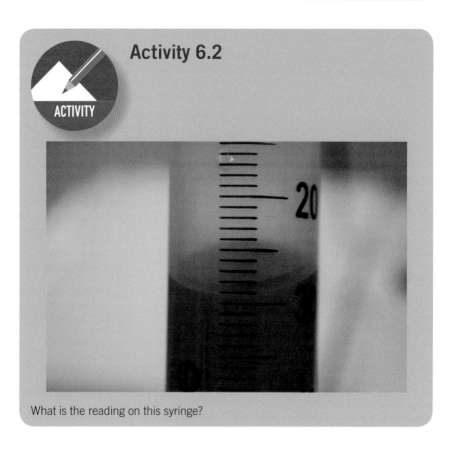

What is the reading on this syringe?

Practice reading the meniscus levels of medications in syringes and medicine pots: always read the lowest level of the curve, and always hold the container at eye level, on a flat surface, to obtain an accurate reading.

KEY POINTS

- Looking at syringes, including the oral syringe.
- Looking at injection needle gauge sizes and choosing the correct gauge size for injections.
- Understanding the meniscus effect.

USEFUL WEB RESOURCES

http://www.bnf.org/bnf/bnf/current/104945.htm

You will need to register to access the bnf site (but registration is free)
www.testandcalc.com/quiz/index.asp

Chapter 7
. . . .
DISPLACEMENT VALUES

Calculation Skills for Nurses, Second Edition. Claire Boyd.

LEARNING OUTCOMES

By the end of this chapter you will have an understanding of the displacement value when reconstituting drugs.

Paediatric Care
Relating to the care of infants, children and adolescents.

Neonatal Care
Relating to the care of newborn babies.

Some drugs, such as those needing to be freeze-dried to a powder for storage, require reconstitution with liquid prior to being administered. When dissolved in the liquid, the powder will take up space and will have to be added to the final volume when drawn up into a syringe; this additional volume must be taken into account when thinking about how much liquid to draw into the syringe. Displacement values come into play when less than a whole ampoule or vial needs to be reconstituted. This is a frequent occurrence in paediatric and neonatal care.

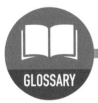

Reconstituting Drugs
Reconstitution refers to building up again; to reconstruct, to restore something to its original state by adding water.

Amoxicillin
Amoxicillin is an antibiotic of the penicillin type.

Let me show you an example. . .

To give a dose of 125 mg amoxycillin from a 250 mg vial:

- the displacement value for amoxycillin 250 mg is 0.2 mL;
- if you add 4.8 mL of fluid, you will then have a total of 5 mL in the vial (4.8 mL + 0.2 mL displacement value), giving you 250 mg in 5 mL;
- therefore, to administer 125 mg, you will need to administer 2.5 mL of the solution.

Let's Explain this Another Way

A patient is prescribed 1.5 g ceftazidime BD (which means twice a day), administered as a bolus. You have been provided with a 2 g vial, which needs to be reconstituted (with water for injection, or WFI) to make a total volume of 10 mL. The displacement value is 1.5 mL/2 g vial.

To make up to a total of 10 mL, you need to add 8.5 mL WFI. This is because the displacement value takes up 1.5 mL (10 mL – 1.5 mL = 8.5 mL).

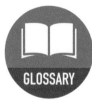

Ceftazidime
Ceftazidime is a cephalosporin antibiotic used to treat enterobacterial infections.

Bolus Injection
The injection of a drug in a single volume

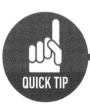

This can be expressed as 'volume to be added equals dilutant volume minus displacement value'.

Now that you have a volume of 10 mL, how many millilitres of this solution will you draw up to administer 1.5 g of the drug?

If you were to draw all the liquid from the ampoule, you would have 10 mL in the syringe. However, you do not want this full amount because the vial contained 2 g, and the prescribed dose is 1.5 g. So, use my formula to find out how much of this liquid you would need to draw out to make the prescribed dose of 1.5 g.

$$\text{Volume of drug to be given} = \frac{\text{what you want}}{\text{what you've got}} \times \text{volume}$$

$$\frac{1.5\,g}{2\,g} \times 10\,mL = 7.5\,mL$$

So, 7.5 mL contains the required amount ordered on the prescription: 1.5 g.

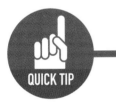

This means that if I had been asked to reconstitute a drug in 4 mL WFI, this is the *total* that will be in the syringe at the end, ready for administration, so that's why I don't actually add 4 mL of WFI to the vial.

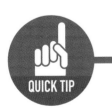

For explanations of Latin abbreviations like BD, and others, see the list at the start of the book.

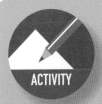

Activity 7.1

1   A patient is prescribed 600 mg of benzylpenicillin. The drug is presented in 600 mg vials, which need to be reconstituted (medic's instructions) in 4 mL of water for injection. Displacement value is 0.4 mL/600 mg. How much water do you add to the vial?

2   A small child has been prescribed 350 mg ceftriaxone IV daily. The drug is presented in 1 g vials and requires reconstituting in water for injection (WFI) to make a total volume of 10 mL. Displacement value is 0.8 mL/g. What volume of WFI needs to be added to the vial to make a total of 10 mL?

3   A 1 gram vial of cefotaxime IV needs to be reconstituted to 4 mL water for injection (WFI). The displacement value is 0.5 mL/g. What volume of WFI do you add to the vial?

4   A vial of flucloxacillin 250 mg needs to be reconstituted in 5 mL WFI. Displacement value = 0.2 mL to every 250 mg vial. What volume of WFI do you add to this vial?

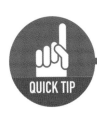

Don't be fooled! There is so much information in these questions – only pull out what you need. They are actually much simpler to answer than you think!

1   **Just subtract 0.4 from 4 mL**
2   **Just subtract 0.8 from 10 mL**
3   **Just subtract 0.5 from 4 mL**
4   **Just subtract 0.2 from 5 mL**

KEY POINTS

- Looking at reconstituting freeze-dried drugs from a powder to a liquid.
- Understanding the importance of displacement when reconstituting drugs.

USEFUL WEB RESOURCES

http://www.bnf.org/bnf/bnf/current/104945.htm

You will need to register to access the bnf site (but registration is free)

Chapter 8

. . . .

DOSAGES ACCORDING TO BODY WEIGHT

Calculation Skills for Nurses, Second Edition. Claire Boyd.
© 2022 John Wiley & Sons Ltd. Published 2022 by John Wiley & Sons Ltd.

LEARNING OUTCOMES

By the end of this chapter you will be familiar with how to titrate drug dosages according to body weight using the 'weight (kg) multiplied by dose' formula.

Some drugs need to be titrated according to a person's body weight. For example, a small child will require a much smaller dose of a drug than a large adult. The formula we can use to titrate the amount is weight (in kg) multiplied by dose:

$$\textbf{Correct dosage} = \textbf{weight}\left(\textbf{kg}\right) \times \textbf{dose}$$

For example, if we had a small lady weighing 55 kg and a 2 mg drug, we could use the above formula, which works out as 55 kg × 2 mg = 110 mg of the drug, either per day or per hour, according to the prescription. A 70 kg patient would require 140 mg of the drug either per day or per hour (that's 70 × 2).

Titration

The process of determining the concentration of a substance in solution to be administered to individuals according to body weight.

GLOSSARY

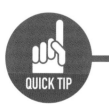

This formula is used a lot in paediatric patients, neonates, critical care and the elderly.

It is always important to get your answer checked.

QUICK TIP

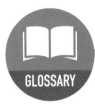

Critical Care

Critical care relates to the specialised care of patients whose conditions are life-threatening and who require comprehensive care and monitoring.

Let's work through some examples:

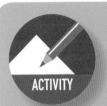

Activity 8.1

A Practice Nurse needs to check the prescriptions for the following patients before administering the medication. Are they correct?

	DOSE PRESCRIBED	DOSE	PATIENT'S WEIGHT
1	116 mg	8 mg/kg/day	15.5 kg
2	9906 mg	12 mg/kg/day	82.55 kg
3	450 mg	7.5 mg/kg/day	60 kg
4	4290 mg	10 mg/kg/day	42.9 kg
5	33.5 mg	2.5 mg/kg/day	14.6 kg
6	711.2 mg	8 mg/kg/day	88.9 kg

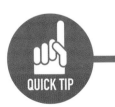

It does not matter which way round you use the formula – it works both ways when answering the questions above:

**Weight (kg) × Dose OR/
Dose × Weight (kg)**

Ready for some more?

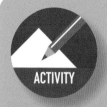

Activity 8.2

1   A patient weighing 70 kg is prescribed 10 mg/kg/h of a drug. How many milligrams per hour of the drug does the patient need? Note that h means hour.
2   Paracetamol is prescribed as 10 mg/kg daily and can be given every 8 hours. How much would you give to a baby weighing 2.5 kg, both daily and every 8 hours?
3   Ranitidine is prescribed as 2 mg/kg. How many milligrams will be prescribed to a baby weighing 0.57 kg?

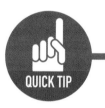

QUICK TIP

If baby's weight is in grams, you will need to convert to kilograms to fit the formula.

4   A drug is prescribed as 30 mg/kg. The patient weighs 48 kg. What dose should be given? If this dose is to be administered in three equal doses daily, how much is given in each dose?

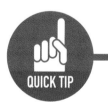

QUICK TIP

Remember drugs may be administered:

OD = once a day
BD = twice a day
TDS = three times a day
QDS = four times a day

Some drugs may need to be administered more frequently than this (e.g., hourly), or less frequently than this (e.g., once every 3 months).

5   A 15-kg child is prescribed a drug 40 mg/kg/day, four doses daily. Calculate a single dose.
6   A 20-kg child is prescribed a drug 80 mg/kg/day, four doses daily. Calculate a single dose.
7   Flucloxacillin is prescribed as 100 mg/kg/day, four doses daily. The patient weighs 58 kg. Calculate a single dose.
8   A patient weighs 92 kg. A drug is prescribed as 60 mg/kg/day, four doses per day. Calculate a single dose.
9   A patient weighs 35 kg. Capreomycin sulphate is prescribed as 20 mg/kg/ day, three doses per day. Calculate a single dose.
10 A 20-kg child is prescribed 45 mg/kg/day of a drug, four doses per day. Calculate a single dose.

KEY POINTS

- Looking at calculating dosages according to body weight using the formula 'weight (kg) multiplied by dose'.
- Understanding the importance of drug titration.
- Looking at Latin abbreviations for administering drugs.

USEFUL WEB RESOURCES

http://www.bbc.co.uk/schools/gcsebitesize/maths/number/
http://www.bnf.org/bnf/bnf/current/104945.htm

You will need to register to access the bnf site (but registration is free)

Chapter 9

· ·

DRIP RATES AND DRIP-RATE DURATIONS

Calculation Skills for Nurses, Second Edition. Claire Boyd.
© 2022 John Wiley & Sons Ltd. Published 2022 by John Wiley & Sons Ltd.

LEARNING OUTCOMES

By the end of this chapter you should be familiar with working out drip-rate calculations using the formula 'volume divided by time multiplied by drops per millilitres divided by minutes per hour' and drip-rate durations using the formula 'volume divided by rate multiplied by drops per millilitre divided by 60 minutes'.

Some patients require IV hydration in the form of a 'drip', which is administered through a line, known as an administration set. Best practice is always to put these fluids through a pump, but sometimes they can be delivered via gravity, meaning without a pump. Many electronic devices require you to input the amount of liquid you intend to administer divided by the time in hours or minutes, depending on the machine set up. For example, you have 1 litre of 0.9% sodium chloride to be administered over 6 hours: You will need to input 1000 mLs divided by 6 = 166.66 = 167 mLs/hr. More about pumps in Chapter 10, but first let's look at examples for these types of machines:

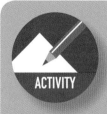

Activity 9.1

ACTIVITY

1 To be administered: ½ litre 5% Dextrose over 2 hours
2 To be administered: 2 litres 0.9% sodium Chloride over 8 hours
3 To be administered: IV antibiotics (made up to 10 mLs) added to 100 mL bag of 0.9% Sodium Chloride over 30 mins
4 To be administered: 1 litre Lactated Ringers solution over 2 hours

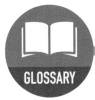

Hartmann's Solution

This is a solution containing sodium chloride, sodium lactate and phosphates of calcium and potassium, used intravenously. May also be called Lactated Ringers solution.

The calculation required for gravity-fed infusions (the manual method for working out the infusion rate), gives us an answer in drops per minute. In order to calculate the rate in drops per minute, the following formula is used:

$$\text{Rate} = \frac{\text{volume}}{\text{time in hours}} \times \frac{\text{drops per millilitre}}{\text{minutes per hour}}$$

Let's break the formula up into parts to make sense of it. The **volume** is the amount that has been prescribed; for example, 1 L of sodium chloride 0.9%. The **time in hours** is also what has been prescribed by the medic, and may be something like 'to be given over 8 hours'.

Minutes per hour is always 60, as there are only 60 minutes in an hour (even in my universe where friends tell me I am in a world of my own)! The **drops per millilitre** depends on the type of fluid being infused and the type of giving set (or administration set) in use. In general. check the infusion set packaging for the flow rate of the set.

Blood administration or standard giving set:

- Blood and 'thick' fluids   15 drops/mL
- Clear fluids   20 drops/mL

Microdrip or paediatric giving set, sometimes referred to as a microdrop burette:

- Clear fluids   60 drops/mL

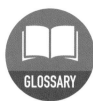

Burette

A burette is a glass or plastic tube with fine graduations and a stopcock at the bottom.

Putting this all together, we work this out as:

Volume amount divided by time in hours multiplied by drops per millilitre (depends on the infusate) divided by minutes per hour (always 60)

When we have worked out our answer, we need to count the 'drip rate', adjusting this accordingly until we get the correct number of drops dripping into the drip-rate chamber.

Let me show you an example...

A patient is to receive 1 L of 5% glucose in 8 hours. Calculate the rate in drops per minute, using a standard giving set (20 drops/mL).

Using the above formula:

$$\text{Rate} = \frac{1000\,\text{mL}}{8\,\text{hours}} \times \frac{20\,\text{drops / mL}}{60\,\text{minutes}} = \frac{1000}{8} \times \frac{20}{60}$$

$$= 41.66$$

$$= 42\,\text{drops per minute}\,(\text{to the nearest drop})$$

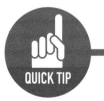

You need to use the rule of 5s to get a whole drop as your answer.

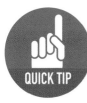

QUICK TIP

Work this out all in one go on your calculator: 1000 divided by 8 multiplied by 20 divided by 60 = 41.666666.

The answer to this question is 41.6, but as we can't count part of a drop, we follow the rule of 5s, and round 41.6 up to the next whole number: in this case 42 drops per minute. When we set up the equipment, we count 42 drops, dripping into the drip chamber: speeding it up, or slowing the drips down using the roller clamp. The end of the administration set gets attached to a cannula on the patient, so that the medication gets delivered straight into the patient intravenously.

ACTIVITY

Activity 9.2

1   1.5 L of sodium chloride has been prescribed to run over 12 hours. Using a standard IV administration set delivering 20 drops/mL, how many drops per minute will the infusion run at?

2   Calculate the following to the nearest whole drop: 420 mL of blood is to be given to a patient over 4 hours using a blood administration set (15 drops/mL).

3   150 mL of Hartmann's solution is prescribed to run over 6 hours. The microdrip administration set delivers 60 drops/mL. How many drops per minute will the infusion be set to run?

4   A patient has been prescribed 350 mL of blood to be administered over 3 hours. Calculate the rate in drops per minute.

5   A patient is to receive half a litre of dextrose 5% over 6 hours. Calculate the rate in drops per minute.

6   A patient has two intravenous lines inserted. One line is running at 25 mL/ hour and the other at 30 mL/hour. What volume of fluid does the patient receive in a 24 hour period?

7 A patient is prescribed 1 L of sodium chloride 0.9% to run over 6 hours. Calculate the drip rate in drops per minute.

8 1.5 L of clear fluid is prescribed to run over 10 hours. Calculate the drip rate in drops per minute.

9 A unit of packed red cells of blood (260 mL) is to be administered over 2 hours. Calculate the drip rate in drops per minute.

10 A unit of 250 mL of packed red blood cells is being administered. Half of this unit has already been transfused. A doctor has requested that the remaining half unit be administered over 1 hour. Calculate the drip rate in drops per minute.

11 A small baby has been prescribed 200 mL of 5% glucose to run over 2 hours through a microdrop administration set. Calculate the drip rate in drops per minute.

12 150 mL of 0.9% saline has been prescribed to run over 4 hours through a microdrop administration set. Calculate the drip rate in drops per minute.

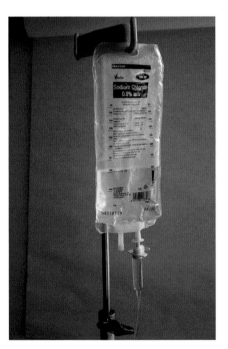

NOTE: when administering blood, or potassium additives to a bag of fluid, a volumetric pump should always be used. This is a specialised piece of machinery with an alarm to alert staff when the fluids have 'gone through' or if air has got into the tubing, etc.

Bags of fluids (such as sodium chloride 0.9%) are best administered via a volumetric pump. This also applies to quantities of fluid over 50 mL. A volumetric pump delivers fluid in whole millilitres per hour, after you have programmed it with the information of how much liquid is to go through and at what time.

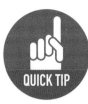

Having a formula makes working out drip rates easy!

DRIP RATE DURATION

It is sometimes necessary to work out how long an infusion will take to complete, or 'go through', before the bag is empty. The formula we use for this is very similar to the drip-rate formula, but as we already know how many drops per minute are going through, this gets added to the formula as 'rate of infusion' or 'drops per minute':

$$\text{Drip} - \text{rate duration} = \frac{\text{volume}}{\frac{\text{rate of infusion}}{\left(\text{drops per minute}\right)} \times \frac{\text{drops per millilitre}}{60\,\text{minutes}}}$$

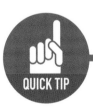

You need to know how to work out these rates manually in case a pump is not available.

It may also be necessary to adjust the rate, using the roller clamp, to speed up or slow down the infusion.

REMEMBER: this formula is for manual application of fluids, as pumps deliver fluids in millilitres per hour.

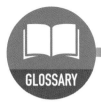

Roller Clamp

A roller clamp is part of the IV administration line that adjusts the drip rate (speeds up or slows down the flow rate).

Let me show you an example...

A patient has received approximately 800 mL of his sodium chloride 0.9% w/v prescription from a 1 L bag of fluid in 6 hours. As this is clear fluids, the administration set delivers 20 drops per millilitre. The fluid was dripping at 42 drops per minute. 'How long has the infusion got left to go?' someone asks. This is how I work out the answer:

First, I look at the bag and estimate that there is 200 mL left to infuse. Then I put the information into my formula:

$$\frac{200}{42} \times \frac{20}{60} = 1.587$$

Which means that there is just over 1½ hours left to infuse these fluids.

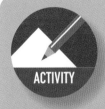

Activity 9.3

1   A patient is to have 3 L of clear fluid in 24 hours. He has received 1500 mL in 8 hours. How many drops per minute are required to correct the infusion?
2   600 mL of fluid is dripping at 20 drops per minute. The IV set delivers 15 drops per millilitre. How long will the infusion take?

3 1000 mL of fluid is dripping at 20 drops per minute. The IV set delivers 15 drops per millilitre. How long will the infusion take?

4 A patient is to have 2 L of clear fluid in 24 hours. She has received 1500 mL in 6 hours. How many drops per minute are required to correct the infusion?

5 Volume of clear fluid = 1000 mL. Rate of infusion = 43 drops per minute. How long will the infusion take?

KEY POINTS

- How to use a formula to work out drip rates on gravity infusions.
- Looking at blood administration sets.
- Looking at standard administration sets.
- Looking at microdrip and burette IV fluid devices.
- How to use a formula to work out drip-rate durations.

USEFUL WEB RESOURCES

http://www.bbc.co.uk/schools/gcsebitesize/maths/number/
http://www.bnf.org/bnf/bnf/current/104945.htm

You will need to register to access the bnf site (but registration is free)

Chapter 10
· ·
SYRINGE DRIVERS
AND PUMPS

Calculation Skills for Nurses, Second Edition. Claire Boyd.
© 2022 John Wiley & Sons Ltd. Published 2022 by John Wiley & Sons Ltd.

LEARNING OUTCOMES

By the end of this chapter you should be familiar with working out calculations in millilitres per hour using the formula 'volume divided by time' and in measuring millimetres per hour.

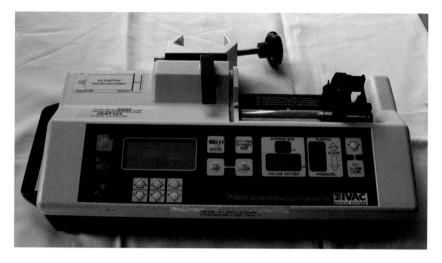

Some drugs, such as heparin and analgesics, need to be administered via specialised machinery, such as a syringe pump, which are sometimes referred to as 'syringe drivers'. These devices deliver set amounts of very concentrated drugs and with low flow rates, usually anything from 0.1 to 99 mL/hour. It is important that anyone using these devices undergoes specialist training, as many different devices are used in clinical areas.

The formula for working out the intravenous infusion rate in millilitres per hour for syringe pumps is:

$$\frac{\text{Infusion rate}}{(\text{mL/hour, pump})} = \frac{\text{amount of fluid}\,(\text{mL})}{\text{infusion time}\,(\text{hours})}$$

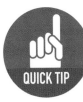

This can be shortened to $\dfrac{\text{volume}}{\text{time}}$

So, if I had 48 mL of fluid in my syringe to be delivered over 24 hours, I would input:

$$\frac{48\,\text{mL}}{24\,\text{hours}} = 2\,\text{mL/hour}$$

Therefore, I would set the machine to deliver 2 mL per hour, and after 24 hours my syringe would be empty.

Now, let's see how you get on with the following questions:

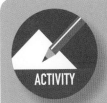

Activity 10.1

1 Mr Smith is prescribed a ***total volume*** of 48 mL of heparin and dilutant to be administered over 24 hours. What is the infusion rate in millilitres per hour? If you get this one wrong, you will know that you have missed the explanations (see above!).
2 An insulin infusion containing 50 units of human Actrapid has been diluted with 50 mL of sodium chloride, which has been running at:

> 3 mL/hour for 2 hours
> 3.5 mL/hour for 3 hours
> 2 mL/hour for 1 hour
> 2.5mL/hour for 1 hour
> 4 mL/hour for 2 hours

How many units of Actrapid insulin in total has the patient received?
3 1 L of normal saline is to be administered over 8 hours. How many millilitres per hour is this?

4 A patient is to receive half a litre of normal saline over 6 hours. How many millilitres an hour should the pump be set?

5 Heparin has been diluted with an infusate to make a total volume of 48 mL in the syringe. This is to be given over 12 hours. At what rate should the infusion pump be set?

6 Over a 12-hour period, a patient is to receive 1 L of dextrose. At what rate should the infusion pump be set?

7 A patient is to receive 24 mL of medication over 12 hours. At what rate should the infusion pump be set?

8 100 mL of metronidazole has been prescribed to run over half an hour. At what rate should the infusion pump be set?

9 80 mL of fluid is to be infused over 30 minutes. At what rate should the infusion pump be set?

10 75 mL of fluid needs to be infused over 20 minutes. Calculate the rate in millilitres per hour.

Metronidazole

Metronidazole is a synthetic anti-microbial drug, used to treat infections.

GLOSSARY

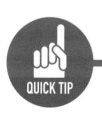

QUICK TIP

Watch out! She's trying to catch us out: did you notice that Question 10 is presented in minutes and the answer needs to be in millilitres per *hour*. Don't forget to multiply the 75 mL by 60 minutes to get the hourly rate.

$$\frac{\text{Volume}\,(\text{mL}) \times 60\,\text{minutes}}{\text{Time}\,(\text{minutes})}$$

This method can be used when infusion times are given in minutes, and when medication has been added to a burette. Do you remember from Chapter 9 that a burette is a microdrip administration set, administered via a volumetric pump? We use this when we need to convert our answer to millilitres per hour.

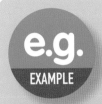

Let me show you an example. . .

Penicillin has been added to a burette to make up a total volume of 40 ml. The infusion time is 20 minutes.

$$\frac{40\,mL \times 60\,minutes}{20\,minutes} = 120\,mL/hour$$

Activity 10.2

Medications have been added to each of these burettes to make a total volume of fluid. Calculate the required pump settings in millilitres per hour.

1   Penicillin added to make a total volume of 50 mL of fluid. To be administered over 20 minutes.
2   Penicillin added to make a total volume of 100 mL of fluid. To be administered over 30 minutes.
3   Flucloxacillin added to make a total volume of 100 mL of fluid. To be administered over half an hour.
4   Vancomycin added to make a total volume of 120 mL of fluid. To be administered over 50 minutes.
5   Gentamicin added to make a total volume of 80 mL of fluid. To be administered over 50 minutes.
6   Ranitidine added to make a total volume of 60 mL of fluid. To be administered over 45 minutes.

Did you notice that the dosage of medication did not have a bearing on our calculations? The drug amount was incorporated into the total volume amount for you, and it is this that we put into the formula. For instance, in Question 1, the penicillin dose was 600 mg, which equated to 5 mL, but you did not have this information, and did not need it to work out the answer in this case. We therefore added this to 45 mL of fluid in the burette to make a total volume of 50 mL.

SYRINGE DRIVERS

These pumps are usually small and compact, can be battery-operated and may be carried by the patient. Some devices deliver continuous subcutaneous infusions, at either an hourly rate (millilitres per hour) or a daily rate (over 24 hours).

Here's an example of an hourly rate prescription:

A patient is prescribed a dose of diamorphine at 2.5 mg/hour. Work out the dose for 24 hours.

2.5 mg/hour for 24 hours = 2.5 mg × 24 hours = 60 mg/24 hours

Here's an example of an hourly rate in millilitres per hour:

The prescription may state that the patient is to receive 60 mg of diamorphine in 24 hours, so no calculation is needed as this is a straightforward dose.

Millimetres Per Hour

Syringe drivers do not rely on the amount of liquid, or volume, in the syringe, but on the length of the column of fluid. The front of the syringe driver should have a millimetre scale, which is used to measure the length of fluid from the upper edge of the plunger to the 'zero' mark at the top of the syringe. So, the size of the syringe is vitally important to the calculation.

If the syringe contains 8 mL of fluid, then the measurement will be 48 mm.

Here's an example of setting the rate in millimetres per hour.

If the prescription is to be delivered over 24 hours, you use the 48 mm (amount of fluid length in the syringe = 8 mL) and divide this by the infusion time in days:

$$\frac{48\,mm}{24\,hours} = 2\,mm/hour$$

Even though 48 mm is not the volume, for these syringe drivers some individuals use the formula:

$$\frac{Volume}{Time}$$

This could be said to be the same as:

$$\frac{Length\,48\,mm}{Time}$$

These calculations are very advanced and will always require double-checking and two individuals to work them out. If you are a student, get involved as a third checker to gain experience. It is always easier to be shown how to make these advanced calculations in the workplace, but let's see how you get on with following my steps.

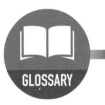

GLOSSARY

Diamorphine
Diamorphine is a powerful heroin opiod drug.

Cyclizine
Cyclizine is an anti-emetic drug often prescribed to treat nausea and/or vomiting.

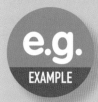

A prescription for diamorphine 20 mg and cyclizine 50 mg is to be given over 24 hours. The syringe driver, which holds a 10 mL syringe, is set to deliver 2 mm/hour. The length of 8 mL in the syringe is measured up as 48 mm. Diamorphine is available in powder form in 10 mg ampoules. Cyclizine is available in ampoules containing 50 mg/2 mL. How is the solution made up?

STEP 1: calculate the total solution required to be delivered at 2 mm/hour.

2 mm / hour × 24 hour = 48 mm

48 mm = 8 mL total solution

STEP 2: calculate the volume of water for injection required to dilute the diamorphlne.

Cyclizine 50 mg = 2 mL

8 mL – 2 mL = 6 mL for the diamorphine

Dilute the 20 mg of dlamorphine with 6 mL of water. Therefore, the syringe contains 8 mL. 6 mL of this is diamorphine and 2 mL of this is cyclizine, making up the total volume of 8 mL. This equates to 48 mm.

Don't worry if you found this too difficult, as you can always come back to look at syringe drivers at a later date. But if you do feel like a challenge, have a go at the next question.

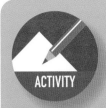

Activity 10.3

1 The prescription is diamorphine 30 mg and cyclizine 50 mg/1 mL, which is to be administered over 24 hours in a syringe driver holding a 10 mL syringe.

   (a) How much water for injection would be required to make up an 8 mL syringe containing cyclizine alone?

   (b) If every 10 mg of diamorphine is to be diluted with 1 mL of water for injection, how much water is required to make the 8 mL syringe of diamorphine and cyclizine together?

   (c) What rate should the syringe driver be set to deliver the 8 mL over 24 hours?

KEY POINTS

- Looking at syringe drivers and pumps.
- How to work out intravenous rates in millilitres per hour.
- How to work out rates according to devices delivering drugs in mm/hour.

USEFUL WEB RESOURCES

www.testandcalc.com/quiz/index.asp

Chapter 11
PAEDIATRIC NURSING

Calculation Skills for Nurses, Second Edition. Claire Boyd.
© 2022 John Wiley & Sons Ltd. Published 2022 by John Wiley & Sons Ltd.

LEARNING OUTCOMES

By the end of this chapter you should be confident and competent in working out drug dosages for neonates and paediatric patients and be aware of the relevance of body weight and body surface area when applying these calculations.

WHAT'S THE DIFFERENCE BETWEEN NURSING CALCULATIONS FOR CHILDREN AND ADULTS?

Many licensed medications have been formulated according to adult dosages, necessitating often complex calculations to administer them to neonates, children and young people. This increases the risk of miscalculation and the potential for harm. Many medications in paediatric nursing are titrated according to body weight (BW) and sometimes even according to body surface area (BSA), incorporating the patient's weight and height into the equation.

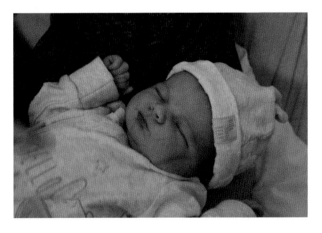

This is also true in adult nursing when dealing with very toxic medications such as chemotherapy drugs.

So, in short, there is not a lot of difference in the actual calculations between adult and paediatric nursing, but in paediatrics more emphasis is placed on certain types of calculation and fluid balance.

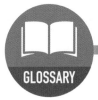

Chemotherapy Drugs

Chemotherapy drugs are cell-killing drugs and growth inhibitors used in the treatment of cancer.

WORKING OUT DRUG DOSAGES

The formulas used in adult nursing fit very well in the paediatric branch of nursing, as it is the digits that are relevant when inputting these figures into the formulas.

$$\text{Number of tablets or capsules required} = \frac{\text{what your want}}{\text{what you've got}}$$

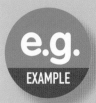

Let me show you an example. . .

A small child has been prescribed 100 mg of fluconazole (what you want), which comes in 50 mg capsules (what you've got). If we use the mathematical approach of 'bundling':

50 mg + 50 mg = 100 mg

We can see that two capsules are required, as two lots of 50 mg make 100 mg. Or we can get used to using the formula, which will come into its own when things start to get more complicated:

$$\frac{100\,\text{mg}}{50\,\text{mg}} = 2\,\text{capsules}$$

WORKING OUT WEIGHT CONVERSIONS

We need to be absolutely confident that any dose of medication we are giving to our patient is a safe dose and for this to be achieved we often need to know the weight of our little patient and may need to undertake some conversions.

Remember:

1 kg = 2.2 pounds (lb)
14 pounds (lb) = 1 stone
16 ounces (oz) = 1 pound (lb)

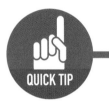

QUICK TIP

You need to know how to convert between imperial and metric units, as parents may ask for their newborn baby's weight in pounds and ounces (the imperial units) if initially given in metric units (kilograms).

e.g.

EXAMPLE

Let me show you an example. . .

A young child weighs 1 stone 6 lb and you need to work out the metric measure:

STEP 1: first you will need to change the weight into *pounds* by multiplying the stones by 14.

1 stone 6 lb $= (1 \times 14) + 6$ **pounds** $= 20$ **pounds in total**

STEP 2: then you need to convert the pounds into kilograms by dividing by 2.2.

20 pounds / 2.2 $= 9.09$ **kg**

So, the child weighs just over 9 kg.

If you need to convert metric units into imperial units, you will need to approach it this way.

A newborn baby weighs 2.8 kg and the parents want to tell their family how much the baby weighs in pounds and ounces.

STEP 1: first you will need to change the kilograms into pounds:

$1 kg = 2.2 lb$

$2.8 kg = 2.2 \times 2.8 = 6.16 lb$

STEP 2: if I wanted to be more accurate, I would take the 0.16 and convert these into ounces.

$1 lb = 16 oz$

So, 0.16 lb × 16 oz = 2.56 oz. Therefore, this little baby weighs 6 lb 3 oz (to the nearest ounce).

WORKING OUT FLUID BALANCE CALCULATIONS

Correct fluid balance calculations are vital in paediatric nursing, as feeds, drug volumes and hydration fluids all need to be within the total fluid allowance of the individual baby or child for their little bodies. A typical calculation may be as follows.

Let me show you an example...

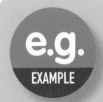

A child weighing 12 kg is prescribed 75% of maintenance fluid over 24 hours. According to local policy, 100% maintenance for a 12 kg child equates to 45 mL/hour. The child is currently receiving drugs at 5 mL/hour by continuous infusion and 10 mL of other drugs administered by injection every 8 hours. What is the amount of feed that can be given every hour?

This is how I would approach this calculation:

STEP 1: add up all the volume of drugs given per hour: 5 mL/hour + 10 mL every 8 hours. I will need to break this 10 mL up to find how much this works out in every hour: 10 mL divided by 8 hours = 1.25 mL/hour.

Total volume of drugs = 5 mL / hour + 1.25 mL / hour = 6.25 mL / hour

STEP 2: now I need to work out what 75% of 45 mL is:

$$\frac{75}{100} \times 45 = 33.75\,\text{mL}$$

This is saying that 100% = 45 mL and 75% = 33.75 mL.

STEP 3: so, now I know that 33.75 mL is the hourly fluid allowance for this child, but, minus the drugs:

33.75 mL − 6.25 mL = 27.5 mL

Therefore, the total amount of feed that our young patient requires is 27.5 mL per hour.

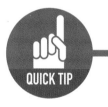

QUICK TIP

For neonatal and paediatric patients, it is very important to be accurate with the volumes given.

WORKING OUT FLUID DRUG CALCULATIONS

$$\frac{\text{Volume of drug}}{\text{to be given}} = \frac{\text{what you want}}{\text{what you've got}} \times \text{volume}$$

Again, this is exactly the same formula for working out fluid doses for injection, syrups, suspensions, etc.

NOTE: remember to always check that the prescription dose and how the drug is presented are both in the same units, or you will need to convert them to the same.

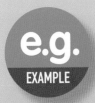

Let me show you an example. . .

A child is prescribed 2.5 mg orally of diazepam. It is presented as 2 mg in 5 mL of suspension. How much do you give?

$$\frac{2.5\,\text{mg}}{2\,\text{mg}} \times 5\,\text{mL} = 6.25\,\text{mL}$$

DRUG DOSAGES ACCORDING TO BODY WEIGHT

$$\text{Correct dosage} = \text{weight}\,(\text{kg}) \times \text{dose}$$

This is where we titrate the drug dose according to the baby's or child's body weight, which we addressed in Chapter 8. However, a whole dose may need to be broken down into doses to be given 2, 4, 6, 8 or 12 hours apart.

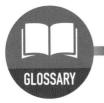

Diazepam
Diazepam is a tranquilizing muscle-relaxant drug used mainly to relieve anxiety.

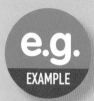

Let me show you an example...

A child weighing 29 kg has been prescribed ampicillin 80 mg/kg/day, which is to be given as four doses per day. How much do you administer in a single dose?

Using the above formula, I can work out that 29 kg × 80 mg/kg/day = 2320 mg/day. This is the amount that the child needs to receive per day, so I will need to divide this into 4 for a single dose:

2320 / 4 = 580 mg / dose

Therefore, the child needs to receive 580 mg of the drug four times a day, as per the prescription.

DOSAGES ACCORDING TO SURFACE AREA

Body surface area (BSA) is literally the surface area of the human body. It can be worked out using an individual's height and weight measurements and may be used to calculate drug dosages and fluid intake very accurately. It is more commonly used when calculating chemotherapy doses, due to their toxicity, and in paediatric prescribing. Other influential factors when calculating BSA include the age and gender of the individual.

The most commonly used simplified formula to determine BSA is the Mosteller, which is expressed as follows:

Body surface area: the square root of product of the weight in kilograms multiplied by the height in centimetres divided by 3600. The result is in square metres.

Or how I express this:

$$BSA\left(m^2\right) = \sqrt{\frac{height\left(cm\right) \times weight\left(kg\right)}{3600}}$$

Then, to calculate BSA using this formula, I get my calculator: I put in the height (or length) of the child in centimetres and multiply it by the weight of the child in kilograms. I then divide the result by 3600 (don't worry about where the 3600 comes from, just go with it). When I have an answer I press the square root button on my calculator to get the BSA in square metres (m²).

However, many people use a scale called a nomogram to estimate BSA, although it is considered to be much less accurate that the Mosteller formula. The figure shows a nomogram for calculating BSA in infants. There are separate nomograms for infants, children and adults.

Let me show you how to use the nomogram. First, get a ruler or something with a straight edge. If we want to find the BSA of an infant with a length of 70 cm and a weight of 32 kg we place the straight edge on the height scale at 70 cm and across to the weight scale at 32 kg. The straight edge crosses the surface area scale at approximately 0.78. This means that the BSA is 0.78 m². Try this out for yourself on the nomogram.

Now, put the same details into the Mosteller formula. You will need a calculator for this exercise, one with a square root button:

$$\boxed{\sqrt{}}$$

$$\frac{Height \times weight}{3600} = \frac{70\,cm \times 32\,kg}{3600} =$$

Using your calculator, input:

$$70 \times 32 = 2240/3600 = 0.62$$

Then find the square root, or press the square root button on your calculator, and you get 0.79 m².

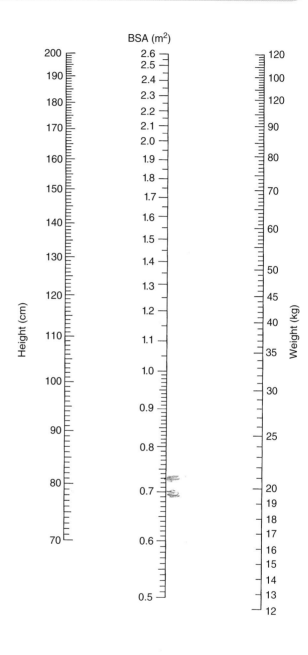

Activity 11.1

Now, let's put everything into practice and try a few questions. If you get stuck, just go back to the section dealing with that particular question and follow the steps again. All the answers, with the workings out, are given in the Answers section at the end of the book. Don't peep: have a go first!

1. Oral paracetamol 50 mg is prescribed. It is presented as 120 mg in 5 mL. What volume do you draw up?
2. Oral phenobarbital (phenobarbitone) 35 mg is prescribed. It is available as 15 mg in 5 mL. What volume would you give?
3. Erythromycin 30 mg/kg/day is prescribed to a child weighing 12 kg. The child is to receive this medication over four doses per day. Calculate a single dose.
4. A child weighing 36 kg has been prescribed flucloxacillin 80 mg/kg/day over four doses. Calculate a single dose.
5. A child weighs 2 stone 8 lb. Work out the metric weight.
6. A child weighs 6.10 kg. Work out the imperial weight.
7. A child weighs 12 kg and is prescribed 75% of maintenance fluid over 24 hours (100% maintenance for a 12 kg child is 45 mL/hour). The child is presently receiving medication by continuous infusion at 2 mL/hour, 8 mL of another medication every 8 hours and 2 mL of a third drug every 6 hours. What is the amount of feed that this child can receive every hour?
8. Digoxin 125 micrograms is prescribed. The drug is presented as 0.5 mg in 2 mL. Calculate the volume you need to draw up.
9. Pethidine 20 mg is prescribed. The drug is presented as 50 mg in 1 mL. Calculate the volume to be drawn up.
10. Use the nomogram shown in this chapter to find the body surface area (BSA) of a child weighing 16.0 kg with a length of 94 cm.
11. Use the nomogram to find the BSA of a child with a length of 95 cm and a weight of 14.0 kg.
12. Using the Mosteller formula, work out the BSA of a child weighing 14.0 kg and with a length of 87 cm.

KEY POINTS

- Understanding weight conversions.
- Understanding fluid balance calculations.
- Looking at the calculation of body surface area using a nomogram.
- Looking at the calculation of body surface area using the Mosteller formula.

USEFUL WEB RESOURCES

http://cmbi.bjmu.cn/servese/clinical/nomogram/nomochil.htm

BNF for children: https://bnfc.nice.org.uk

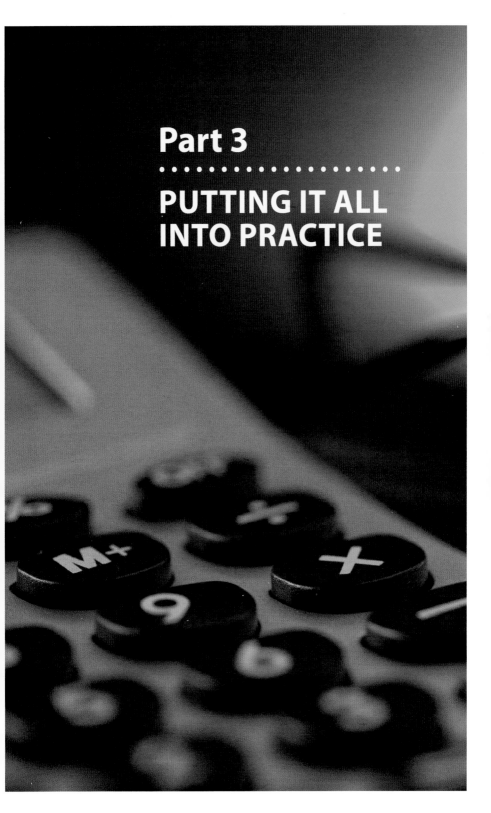

Part 3
. . . .
PUTTING IT ALL INTO PRACTICE

Chapter 12
....
FLUID CHARTS

Calculation Skills for Nurses, Second Edition. Claire Boyd.
© 2022 John Wiley & Sons Ltd. Published 2022 by John Wiley & Sons Ltd.

LEARNING OUTCOMES

By the end of this chapter you should have a working knowledge of fluid charts and the importance of fluid balance.

A fluid chart is a record of the amounts of fluids a patient has taken in during a day (i.e., drinks and any other fluids, such as 5% dextrose saline via the IV route) and the patient's fluid output (i.e., urine, vomit, etc.). The output total is subtracted from the intake total and the balance is recorded. When intake is greater than output, a positive balance is recorded, but if intake is less than output, the fluid balance is recorded as being negative.

Appendix 1 shows a typical fluid chart

Accurately monitoring a patient's fluid balance is crucial to a patient's well-being, as the body works within very narrow parameters and is always striving for homeostasis. In short, any water loss needs to be replaced for the body's water volume to remain constant.

In males, total body fluid constitutes approximately 60% of the body weight. In females, total body fluid constitutes approximately 52% of total body weight.

Too little fluid in the body, perhaps due to excessive diarrhoea, vomiting or sweating due to fever, is known as hypovalemia. Too much fluid, perhaps caused by over-infusion of intravenous fluids, congestive cardiac failure or renal failure, is known as hypervalemia. It takes just a small amount of variation from the norm to cause havoc within the body:

- a reduction of 5% causes thirst
- a reduction of 8% causes illness
- a reduction of 10% can cause death.

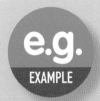

Let me show you an example. . .

Here's how to work out a person's fluid balance.

Today I have drunk:

* two cups of coffee: 150 mL per cup,
* four cups of tea: 150 mL per cup,
* one cola: 300 mL,
* one bottle of spring water: 500 mL.

I add all this up, which equals 1700 mL. This is my input.

I went to the toilet to pass urine four times throughout the day, passing 400 mL, 600 mL, 200 mL and 450 mL. I add this up, which equals 1650 mL. This is my output.

I then subtract my output from my input = 1700 mL – 1650 mL = 50 mL. This is my fluid balance, pretty good! Note that we tend to look at longer periods to see trends for fluid balance.

Fluid Balance
Fluid balance relates to the difference between the amount of fluid taken into the body and the amount excreted or lost.

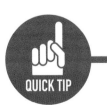

The 24-hour fluid record chart generally starts at 08.00 and the final tally gets totted up at 07:00, just before the early shift may start for the day.

Activity 12.1

Mrs Maxwell has had a cup of tea (150 mL) at the following times:

08:00	150 mL
10:00	150 mL
12:00	150 mL
14:00	150 mL
18:00	150 mL
22:00	150 mL

Mrs Maxwell has also had a blackcurrant drink (188 mL) at 13:00 and a small cola (150 mL) at 17:00. Finally, at 06:00 Mrs Maxwell drank 1500 mL of water from her water jug.

Mrs Maxwell has a urinary catheter in place which was emptied at 16:00; the amount was 750 mL.

Plot all these amounts on the input part of the fluid balance chart (see Appendix 1).

What is Mrs Maxwell's fluid balance? (That's input amount *minus* output amount.)

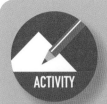

Activity 12.2

Work out the total input, total output and fluid balance for these patients.

1 **Intake**
IV fluids = 1500 mL
Oral fluids = 75 mL
Output
Urine = 1020 mL
Vomit = 75 mL
Wound drainage = 15 mL

2 **Intake**
IV fluids = 850 mL
Oral fluids = 275 mL
Output
Urine = 525 mL
Vomit = 60 mL
Wound drainage = 50 mL

3 **Intake**
Oral fluids = 950 mL
Output
Urine = 500 mL
Liquid diarrhoea = 400 mL

4 **Intake**
Oral fluids = 1750 mL
Output
Urine = 500 mL

5 **Intake**
IV fluids = 1 L
Oral fluids = 150 mL
Output
Wound Leak = 50 mL
Vomit = 50 mL

6 **Intake**
Oral fluids = 500 mL
Output
Urine = 900 mL

Children's fluid balance is calculated the same way as for adults but obviously for much smaller amounts. With babies and very young children wearing nappies and those who need to wear incontinence pads and who require fluid balance records, these nappies and pads will need to be weighed. A rule of thumb is that 1 g = 1 mL.

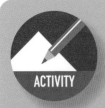

Activity 12.3

1   Baby A had a wet nappy weighing 137 g. The dry nappy weighed 18 g. What is the amount recorded on the fluid balance chart?

2   Baby B has had his wet nappy subtracted from his dry nappy and this has been recorded on the fluid balance chart. What is his total fluid balance?

Input: 120 mLs milk	Output: 50 mLs urine
50 mLs water	55 mLs urine
80 mLs milk	100 mLs urine
18 mLs milk	60 mLs urine
50 mLs water	20 mLs urine
70 mLs milk	75 mLs urine
100 mLs milk	55 mLs urine

KEY POINTS

- Looking at fluid charts.
- Looking at fluid balance.

USEFUL WEB RESOURCES

www.bbc.co.uk/schools/ks2bitesize/maths/number/addition/read1.shtml

www.bbc.co.uk/schools/k2bitesize/maths/number/subtraction/read1.html

Chapter 13

· · · · · · · · · · · · · · · · · · · ·

MALNUTRITION UNIVERSAL SCREENING TOOL (MUST) ASSESSMENT

Calculation Skills for Nurses, Second Edition. Claire Boyd.
© 2022 John Wiley & Sons Ltd. Published 2022 by John Wiley & Sons Ltd.

LEARNING OUTCOMES

By the end of this chapter you should have a working knowledge of the Malnutrition Universal Screening Tool (MUST) assessment.

MUST, or Malnutrition Universal Screening Tool, is a five-step screening tool to identify *adults* (not children) who are malnourished, at risk of malnutrition (undernutrition) or obese. It also includes management guidelines which can be used to develop a care plan. Take a few minutes to look at the MUST assessment guidelines in Appendix 2.

Now let me show you how to use the MUST assessment by working through the steps.

Step 1   First I work out the body mass index (BMI) of my patient, in this case a gentleman who measures 1.76 m in height and weighs 95 kg. Using these figures on the chart, I find that this equates to a BMI of 31 kg/m^2, and score of zero.

Step 2   I look to see if there has been any unplanned weight loss in the past 3 to 6 months. There is none for my make-believe patient, so the score is another zero.

Step 3   For this part of the process I look to see if there are any acute diseases present, and as there are none for my patient, the score is zero.

Step 4   This next part requires me to add up all my scores to establish the overall risk of malnutrition and, as I have a zero, the MUST score is deemed to be low risk and so I follow the management guidelines for low-risk patients.

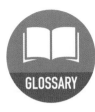

Malnutrition
Lack of adequate nutrition.

Malnourished
Suffering from malnutrition.

Obese
Excess body fat or overweight.

NOTE: even though this make-believe patient is obese, this does not rule him out from malnutrition. He may be big, but his diet may be very poor nutritionally. It is often difficult to recognize malnutrition in patients who are overweight or obese.

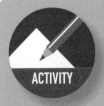

Activity 13.1

Work through the five MUST steps:

Step 1 Dennis Langley is 85 years old. He is 5 feet 5 inches in height and weighs 85 kg. What is his BMI score, and his MUST score for Step 1?

Step 2 Four months ago, Dennis' wife died and he lost some weight, but less than 5%. What is his MUST score for Step 2?

Step 3 Dennis has stopped eating and is drinking very little: this has got worse over the last 5 days. What is his MUST score or Step 3?

Step 4 What is his overall risk of malnutrition score?

Step 5 What is his management strategy?

KEY POINTS

- How to use the Malnutrition Universal Screening Tool (MUST) to identify adults who are malnourished, at risk of malnutrition or obese.

USEFUL WEB RESOURCES

http://www.bapen.org.uk

Chapter 14

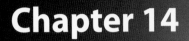

NATIONAL EARLY WARNING SCORE (NEWS 2) ASSESSMENT

Calculation Skills for Nurses, Second Edition. Claire Boyd.
© 2022 John Wiley & Sons Ltd. Published 2022 by John Wiley & Sons Ltd.

LEARNING OUTCOMES

By the end of this chapter you should have a working knowledge of the National Early Warning Score (NEWS 2) assessment.

NEWS 2 is the latest version, from the Royal College of Physicians, of the early warning patient observation chart. The front page of the NEWS 2 chart can be seen in Appendix 3, but for the full version of this document and larger print version, it is recommended that you visit the Royal College of Physicians website – details at the end of this chapter. The NEWS 2 observation chart aims to identify the deteriorating patient or nursing home resident, due to the fact that patients/residents often exhibit abnormalities in their vital signs over a period of hours. It also gives directions on what to do with the information you have collected.

There are six vital signs (or physiological measurements) that are recorded in the order of A, B, C, D, E: on the chart. The NEWS assessment can be used in conjunction with the Early Patient Assessment and Response assessment (known as EPAR), or the ABCDE.

You may want to look at Appendix 3 at this point if you have not already done so:

1.   **A & B = Respiration Rate**

2.   **A & B = Oxygen Saturation**

3.   **C = Systolic Blood Pressure**

4.   **C = Pulse Rate**

5.   **D = Level of consciousness or new confusion**

6.   **E = Temperature**

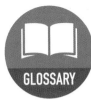

Systolic Blood Pressure

The systolic blood pressure is the pressure exerted on the arterial walls due to the contraction of the heart.

The NEWS 2 chart can be used on:

- All adult in-patients (and care home residents)
- Occasionally children on adult wards
- Pregnant mothers up to 20 week

There are adapted NEWS 2 charts for use with patients requiring neurological observations (with the Glasgow Coma Scale incorporated into the chart), maternity (for pregnant women over 20 weeks' gestation), children, babies and neonates, and patients requiring end of life care.

Neurological Observation

A neurological observation is a collection of information with regard to the central nervous system (the brain and spinal cord).

The NEWS 2 chart is brightly coloured, whereby each vital sign generates a score of 0–3.

- A figure plotted in the white zone of the chart generates a score of 0
- A figure plotted in the yellow zone of the chart generates a score of 1
- A figure plotted in the orange zone of the chart generates a score of 2
- A figure plotted in the red zone of the chart generates a score of 3

Once all the vital signs have been collected, we are directed what to do with this information:

- A total score of 0 directs that we should continue monitoring the patient for a minimum of 12 hours
- A total score of 1–4 directs that we should continue monitoring the patient for a minimum of 4–6 hourly
- A score of 3 in a single parameter directs us to continue monitoring the patient once hourly and to inform the Nurse-in-Charge and the Doctor
- A score of 5 or more directs that we should continue monitoring the patient once hourly and to obtain an urgent medical review
- A total score of 7 or more directs us to perform continuous monitoring of vital signs and to obtain an Emergency medical assessment.

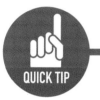

QUICK TIP

It should be noted that we can still use our own clinical judgement, even if the chart does not yet trigger the early warning responses.

You may be wondering why this book contains a chapter on NEWS 2. The simple answer is that this system asks the assessor to add up the scores of the person being assessed and it never ceases to amaze me, in the often frantic clinical areas, how often we add these scores up wrongly, which in turn can affect the treatment and outcome of the patient. Part of the NEWS 2 remit is the timeliness of the response – in short, this system is designed to save lives and a simple miscalculation can have severe repercussions on the patient's well-being. To be fair, some aspects of the chart can be somewhat confusing to the novice, namely the oxygen scales and the D and E aspects of the assessment.

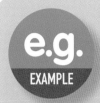

The D part of the A–E assessment:

Disability not only includes the level of consciousness or new confusion but should also include assessment of diuresis, drugs and diabetes (i.e., monitoring blood glucose). However, only the level of consciousness/new confusion is plotted on the chart.

The D part of the assessment assesses the patient using 'ACVPU' and Alert can be used on patients with a usual level of delirium as this may be their norm.

The E part of the A–E assessment:

Temperature is only one aspect of the E for 'Environment' A–E assessment, as it should also include Exposure to assess for bleeding and areas of concern on the patient's body.

Level of Consciousness

There are five recordings for the Neuro response:

1. A = Alert

2. C = New Confusion

3. V = Patient only responding to verbal stimuli

4. P = Patient only responding to painful stimuli

5. U = Patient unresponsive

Alert scores a zero, whilst all other responses score a 3 and necessitate immediate review by the medical team.

Oxygen

Part of the A and B section on the chart assesses the oxygen saturation using two different target scales:

Scale 1 is used for patients who are not at risk of hypercapnic failure.

Scale 2 is used for patients with or AT HIGH RISK of hypercapnic failure.

Only a Doctor, Nurse Practitioner or Specialist Nurse from the Respiratory team can generally authorize the use of scale 2.

An extra score of 2 is added for patients requiring supplemental oxygen. Also, the code for any oxygen giving device should be written in:

A	NC	SM	RM	VM	TM	CH	HH	CP	BP	HFNO
Air	Nasal Cannulae	Simple Mask	Reservoir Mask	Venturi Mask	Tracheostomy Mask	Cold Humidified	Heated Humidified	CPap	BiPap	High Flow Nasal Oxygen

GLOSSARY

Hypercapnic Failure

Hypercapnic respiratory failure means that there is too much carbon dioxide in the blood, e.g., chronic obstructive pulmonary disease (COPD).

If we look at the NEWS 2 chart in Appendix 3, we can see how for scale 1, the scores of 0–3 are plotted on the chart for the patient's oxygen assessments:

96% = scores 0

94–95% = scores 1

92–93% = scores 2

≤ 91% = scores 3

Once we have added up all our patient's assessments, we then need to know what to do with this information. This is where the 'Response' part kicks in, as the full document gives directions on frequency of monitoring and clinical response! It should also be noted that the NEWS 2 chart also assesses the patient's pain score, monitoring frequency, nausea score, etc.

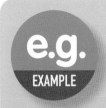

Let me show you an example on how to use the NEWS 2 chart:

1 First, I obtain my patients respiratory rate, which on this occasion is 32 breaths per minute, which generates a score of 2.

2 Next, I look at my patient's oxygen levels and see whether the Doctor admitting my patient is on scale 1 or scale 2, and whether the patient is breathing room air or receiving oxygen. If so, look at which device they are receiving this supplementary oxygen from and write this on the chart, remembering to add 2 to the NEWS score. However, on this occasion, the patient is on Scale 1 so I cross out the Scale 2 section on the chart to avoid any confusion. My patient's oxygen saturations are 94% generating a score of 1.

3 I look at the Blood Pressure part on the chart and record my patients systolic blood pressure as 198 (only the systolic reading is recorded, not the diastolic). This generates a score of 0.

4 Next, I obtain the Heart Rate, which is 81 beats per minute giving me a score of 0.

5 Then I assess my patient and establish that they are fully alert, giving me a score of 0.

6 Next comes the recording of the patient's temperature, which is 37.9 degrees Celsius, giving me a score of 0.

7 Only when I have input all the sections can I add up all my scores. It will mess up the results if I do not fill in all the vital signs sections: 2 + 1 + 0 + 0 + 0 + 0 = 3.

Now have a go at working out four assessments for yourself.

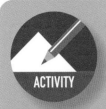

Activity 14.1

Using the NEWS 2 in Appendix 3, work out the score for Mrs Eunice Yonder.

Eunice is 62 years old and has been admitted to hospital due to shortness of breath and difficulty breathing. Her observations on admittance are:

> Respiratory Rate: 30 breaths per minute
> Scale 1 oxygen saturations
> Sp02: 95% on oxygen therapy via nasal spigs
> Blood Pressure: 165/80
> Heart Rate: 90 beats per minute
> ACVPU: Alert
> Temperature: 37.9 Degrees Celsius
> What is her NEWS 2 score?

Activity 14.2

Using the NEWS 2 in Appendix 3, work out the score for Mr Maynard. Mr Maynard is 75 years old and has been admitted to hospital due to severe abdominal pain. His observations on admittance are:

> Respiratory Rate: 18 breaths per minute
> Scale 1 oxygen saturations
> Sp02: 98% on air
> Blood Pressure: 115/72
> Heart Rate: 82 beats per minute
> ACVPU: Alert
> Temperature: 36.9 Degrees Celsius
> What is his NEWS 2 score?

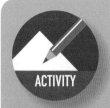

Activity 14.3

Work out the NEWS 2 score:

RR: 24
O2 Sats: 96%
Scale 1
Oxygen Therapy: Air
BP: 105/50
Pulse: 120 bpm
ACVPU: Alert
Temp: 38.1 Degrees Celsius

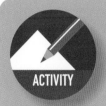

Activity 14.4

Work out the NEWS 2 score:

RR: 25 bpm
O2 Sats 94%
Scale 1
Oxygen Therapy: 35% via venturi mask
BP: 114/70
Pulse: 112 bpm
ACVPU: Alert
Temp: 36 degrees Celsius

KEY POINTS

- How to use the National Early Warning Score (NEWS 2b) tool.
- Understanding the ACVPU assessment.

USEFUL WEB RESOURCES

https://www.rcplondon.ac.uk/projects/outputs/
national-early-warning-score-news

Chapter 15
. . . .
WATERLOW
ASSESSMENT

Calculation Skills for Nurses, Second Edition. Claire Boyd.
© 2022 John Wiley & Sons Ltd. Published 2022 by John Wiley & Sons Ltd.

The Waterlow Pressure Ulcer Prevention/Treatment Policy, or Waterlow risk assessment tool (see Appendix 4), helps us to establish an individual's risk factors for acquiring a pressure ulcer. This forewarns us of the need to utilise specialised equipment such as pressure-relieving mattresses on a patient's bed, and other devices such as cushions and heel guards. The Waterlow tool looks at a patient's medical state, age and gender to work out this score. Using the tool is a very simple matter of using our addition skills and is often carried out by Nursing Assistants in Care Homes.

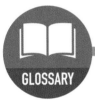

GLOSSARY

Pressure ulcer

A pressure ulcer is an area of skin that has broken down after constant pressure has been applied, or in a combination with shear and/or friction.

e.g.

EXAMPLE

Let me show you an example...

Let me show you how to use the Waterlow assessment tool, using the form shown in Appendix 4.

- I always start off with the age and gender of the patient (don't ask me why, I just do!). So, if I had a male patient this would mean a score of 1 point. If he were aged 72, this would be 3 points. Therefore, in this section (Sex/Age) my patient has scored 4 points for his age and gender.

- Then I go to the start of the assessment tool, to the Build/Weight section and input the details: my patient has an average body mass index, scoring 0 points.
- The next section is the Skin Type and I can see that my patient is quite oedematous or, as he himself describes, 'puffy', so I score him 1 point.
- I have already completed the Sex/Age section, so I move on to the Nutrition section. As my patient has not lost weight recently, I move on to Section C and I learn that my patient has presently lost his appetite, so I score him 1 point.
- I then move on to the Continence section and as my patient has no issues in this area, he gets a score of 0 points.
- The next section I look at is Mobility. He has back pain and this is restricting his mobility, necessitating long periods sitting in a chair; I score him a 3.
- Lastly, I look at Special Risks and as he is a smoker he gets 1 point and he has an Hb value of 4, so he gets 2 points. He is also on high-dose steroids and anti-inflammatory medication for his back pain, for which he gets a further score of 4 points.
- Now I add up the score: $1 + 3 + 0 + 1 + 1 + 0 + 3 + 1 + 2 + 4 = 16$, which equates to a high risk of getting pressure ulcers.

Activity 15.1

ACTIVITY

Using the Waterlow risk assessment tool, work out Molly's Waterlow score. This is done by gathering all the information we have to hand and giving it a score against the assessment tool. For example, Molly immediately gets 2 points just for being female.

Molly Jeffreys is 70 years old and is average weight/build for her height. She has, however, recently lost 9.5 kg in weight, due to 'going off' her food.

Molly has very thin skin, with a lack of subcutaneous tissue. Daisy states that she feels 'very weak' and her mobility is restricted because of this.

After a review by her GP, Molly was found to have a urinary tract infection (and is now wearing a pad and pants due to some urinary incontinence), and also has anaemia.

What is Molly's Waterlow score?

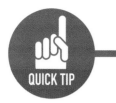

It should be remembered that the Waterlow tool is a dynamic tool meaning that, as patients' conditions change, repeated assessments should be obtained.

Ready for another one?

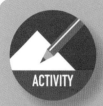

Activity 15.2

David Brennon is being admitted to a Care Home.

Build/Weight for Height: David is obese (above average BMI)

Skin Type Visual Risk Areas: David has oedematous skin

Sex/Age: David is an 82-year-old male

Nutrition: David has not lost weight recently but has a lack of appetite presently

Continence: David has no continence issues

Mobility: David has restricted mobility

Tissue Malnutrition: David is a heavy smoker

Neurological Deficit: None reported or observed

Major Surgery or Trauma: None

Medication: David states that he takes 'large white tablets', which he thinks are some type of steroid. Awaiting his GP surgery to provide this information. Will add 1 to the score in anticipation, to be reviewed once this information has been obtained.

What is David's Waterlow score?

KEY POINT

- How to use the Waterlow risk assessment tool for pressure ulcers.

USEFUL WEB RESOURCES

https://www.thecalculator.co/health/waterlow-score-calculator-1116.html

Chapter 16

· ·

PRESCRIPTION CHARTS

Prescription charts come in many different formats, including electronic, but it should be remembered that they are all legal documents. In most areas there is usually room for two professionals to sign the chart – the person administering the medication and the person checking the prescription and preparation (if required) – especially important for Paediatric areas and in Oncology. Many charts also use the 24-hour clock. If you are not sure about this way of reading and recording time, page xiv can help you. Administering medications from the prescription chart is where all our nursing calculations come into their own.

Remember that to work out how many tablets or capsules, or millilitres of fluid, that we need to administer, we can use the following formulas.

For tablets or capsules:

$$\text{Number of tablets or capsules required} = \frac{\text{what you want}}{\text{what you've got}}$$

For a liquid:

$$\text{Volume of drug to be given} = \frac{\text{what you want}}{\text{what you've got}} \times \text{volume}$$

So, if a medic has prescribed 60 mg of codeine phosphate to a child, every 4–6 hours (maximum dose of 240 mg daily), and the drug is presented in 30 mg tablets, this works out as:

$$\frac{60\,mg}{30\,mg} = 2\ tablets$$

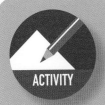

Activity 16.1

Look at the prescription chart and for the drugs listed work out how many tablets, capsules or millilitres of injection the patient requires for each dose, and any special considerations you need to consider. The available formulations of the drugs are given below.

NOTE: when administering drugs, the nurse is required to know about the drug itself (any contra-indications, etc.), and you may wish to use a copy of the British National Formulary while undertaking this activity.

1 Erythromycin: on hand are 250 mg tablets.
2 Aspirin (dispersible tablets): on hand are 75 mg tablets.
3 Tramadol hydrochloride: on hand are 50 mg/mL ampoules for intravenous injection.
4 Propranolol hydrochloride: on hand are 160 mg capsules.
5 Hydroxocobalamin intramuscular injection: on hand are 1 mg/1 mL ampoules.
6 Ketorolac trometamol: on hand are 10 mg/mL ampoules for intravenous injection.

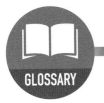

Contra-indication
A condition that makes a particular treatment or procedure inadvisable.

6 hourly	06.00–12.00–18.00–24.00
8 hourly	06.00–14.00–22.00
12 hourly	09.00–21.00

SURNAME (MR/MRS/MISS)		DATE OF BIRTH	UNIT NUMBER
FIRST NAMES		SEX	CONSULTANT
ADDRESS			

REGULAR PRESCRIPTIONS

Date	Drug	Dose	Route	Times of administration	Other directions	Doctor's	Date	Pharm

REGULAR PRESCRIPTIONS

	Date	Drug (approved name – BLOCK CAPITALS)	Dose	Route	6	12	18	24	Other Directions / Duration	Doctor's Signature	Date	Pharm
1	TODAY	ERYTHROMYCIN	500 MG	O	√	√	√	√		A Doctor		
2	TODAY	ASPIRIN (DISPERSIBLE)	300 MG	O		√			AFTER FOOD	A Doctor		
3	TODAY	TRAMADOL HYDROCHLORIDE	75 MG	IV	√	√	√	√	GIVE OVER 2–3 MINS	A Doctor		
4	TODAY	PROPRANOLOL	80 MG	O	√		√			A Doctor		
5	TODAY	HYDROXOCOBALAMIN	1 MG	IM		√			GIVE EVERY 3 MONTHS	A Doctor		
6	TODAY	KETOROLAC TROMETAMOL	35 MG	IV	√		√		ADMINISTER OVER >15 SECONDS	A Doctor		
7												
8												
9												
10												
11												
12												
13												
14												
15												

AS REQUIRED PRESCRIPTIONS

	Date	Drug (approved name – BLOCK CAPITALS)	Dose	Route	Directions	Maximum / Frequency	Doctor's Signature	Date	Pharm
1									
2									
3									
4									
5									
6									
7									
8									
9									

Source: Prescription chart. Reproduced here with permission from North Bristol NHS Trust and University Hospitals Bristol NHS Foundation Trust.

Activity 16.2

A patient's prescription chart shows that the patient is prescribed:

1   soluble aspirin 150 mg
2   diazepam 12.5 mg
3   digoxin 125 micrograms
4   paracetamol 1 gram
5   atenolol 75 mg
6   furosemide 40 mg

Below are the labels on the bottles in the drug trolley, which have all been mixed up. Can you work out the number of tablets or capsules to be administered in each case?

Digoxin	Soluble aspirin	Diazepam
0.25 mg	300 mg	5 mg

Paracetamol	Furosemide	Atenolol
500 mg	40 mg	50 mg

It is also important to understand any abbreviations used on the prescription chart, such as:

- Mcg = micrograms (should be written in full as could be mistaken for mg on the chart)
- PO = By Mouth
- Mg = Milligram
- IM = Intramuscular route
- G = Gram
- IV = Intravenous route
- Kg = Kilogram
- SC = Subcutaneous route
- l = Litre
- PR = Rectal route
- mL = Millilitre

- NJ = Nasojejunal route
- TOP = Topical route
- PV = Vaginal route
- SL = sublingual route
- NEB = By nebuliser
- NG = Nasogastric route
- U = Units

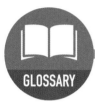

GLOSSARY

Sublingual route
Under the tongue

MARR CHART

In Care Homes, Service Users may use a system called the Medication Administration Record and Request form – known as the MARR chart. Just as there are many different formats of hospital prescription forms, there are many different MARR prescription forms.

Any healthcare professional administering medications to those in his/her care needs to be fully aware as to correct dosages of medication and contra-indications, and never administer a drug just because it has been written on whatever type of prescription form. For example, you would never administer penicillin to an individual whom you know to be allergic to penicillin and most certainly need to have a discussion with the prescriber.

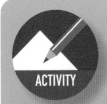

Activity 16.3

A new Service User to Buttercup Meadows Care Home explained to his new care home staff that he self-administers the following prescribed medication, SL, after suffering from a stroke some years previously, from which he made a full recovery, i.e., no left-sided weakness or swallowing difficulties. You make a check of the medication for your own understanding, but something is not quite right. What is it?

MEDICATION	DOSAGE	MODE OF ACTION
Atorvastatin PO	80 mg	Lowers cholesterol
Amlodipine PO	105 mg	Lowers Blood Pressure
Clopidogrel PO	75 mg	For Acute Coronary Syndrome
Ramipril PO	5 mg	Lowers Blood Pressure

KEY POINT

- Administering medications according to a patient's or Service Users prescription chart.
- Understanding abbreviations used on prescription charts.

USEFUL WEB RESOURCES

http://www.bnf.org/bnf/bnf/current/104945.htm

You will need to register to access the bnf site (but registration is free)

Chapter 17
· ·
LOOKING AT BUDGETS

Calculation Skills for Nurses, Second Edition. Claire Boyd.
© 2022 John Wiley & Sons Ltd. Published 2022 by John Wiley & Sons Ltd.

LEARNING OUTCOMES

By the end of this chapter you should have a working knowledge of calculating simple budgets and reading simple charts.

In health care, applying mathematics in the workplace takes many different forms. In this chapter, we will be looking at simple budgets. For example, just knowing that on one ward in a directorate in the hospital they employ five band 6 nurses, all on approximately £32 000 per annum, I know that their annual salaries amount to 6 × £32 000, or £192 000. See if you can work out the training budget for the care home described below.

Activity 17.1

A care home has a budget of £2200 per year for training. The manager would like the home's registered general nurses to have training in venepuncture and adult male catheterisation, which can be received from the local NHS Trust. She would also like the care assistants in the home to undertake training in catheter care.

This year, half of the care assistant staff are due for their Basic Clinical Skills 2-yearly update, again provided by the local NHS Trust.

1   Look at the staff numbers and cost sheet below and state how much this training will cost. Does the care home have enough money to pay for it?

Job title	Number of staff
Registered general nurses	6
Care assistants	24
Customer services	12

Training session	Cost
Venepuncture	£57.50 per person
Adult male urinary catheterisation	£57.50 per person
Catheter care	£57.50 per person
Basic Clinical Skills	£400 per session (no more than 12 individuals in each session)

2   What is the ratio of registered general nurses to care assistants to customer services staff?

Venepuncture
Venepuncture is when a vein is punctured to obtain blood as part of a medical procedure.

As your healthcare career progresses, you may increasingly be required to manage budgets – large departmental ones or smaller cash flows.

You may wish to reacquaint yourselves with earlier sections of this book, for example percentages.

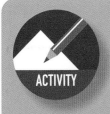

Activity 17.2

1   A Ward Manager on a Mental Health Crisis Unit has a projected annual budget of £600 000. Costs in December are extremely high and are anticipated at 20% of the whole annual costs for December.

2 Tick the correct statement/s:

(a) Costs for all months are equal

(b) Costs in December are £120 000

(c) Costs in December are higher than those in August

(d) Costs in December are £200 000

3 Honesty is a Ward Sister on a Paediatric Ward. Her annual costs are £480 000. If her annual costs increase by 5%, what are her monthly outgoings?

In health care, you may also be expected to interpret data from larger Government budgets.

The chart shows the UK Central Government expenditure for public sector departments in 2016/2017. The revenue to pay for this expenditure is gathered by Her Majesty's Revenue and Customs in the form of taxes.

Expenditure Billion £

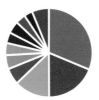

- Social Protection 31.1% = £240bn
- Education 13.2% = £102bn
- Government Debt Interest 5% = £39bn
- Personal Social Service 3.9% = £30bn
- Transport 3.8% = £29bn
- Other (includes EU contribution) 6.3% = £49bn

- Health 18.8% = £145bn
- Defence 6% = £46bn
- Public Order & Safety 4.4% = £34bn
- Housing & Environment 4.4% = £34bn
- Industry -Agriculture & Employment 3.3% = £24bn

Source: Total 2016–2017 Government Expenditure £772 billion.

Activity 17.3

Looking at the UK Government expenditure chart, answer these questions.

1 How much is spent on health care for 2016/2017?
2 What is the largest expenditure for 2016/2017?
3 How much is spent on housing and environment for 2016/2017?
4 What is the financial difference between health, and housing and environment in 2016/2017?

The newly published figures for public sector expenditure for 2019/ 2020 show the following costs for five of these services:

- Social Protection – £275.3 billion
- Health – £164.1 billion
- Education – £92.4 billion
- Defence – £42.2 billion
- Transport – £34.7 billion

If I want to see what the percentage difference for Transport 2016/2017 to 2019/2020 was, I can work it out like this:

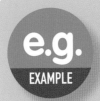

To work out the percentage difference:

Transport 2016/2017 = £29 billion

2019/2020 = £34.7 billion

34.7 – 29 = 5.7

Percentage difference = 5.7

$29 \times 100 = 19.65 = 20\%$ increase in expenditure

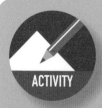

Activity 17.4

1 What is the percentage difference for expenditure on Social Protection from 2016/2017 to 2019/2020?

2 What is the percentage difference for expenditure on Health from 2016/2017 to 2019/2020?

3 What is the total percentage difference for expenditure on Education from 2016/2017 to 2019/2020?

4 What is the total percentage difference for expenditure on Defence from 2016/2017 to 2019/2010?

KEY POINTS

- Looking at budgets.
- How to interpret simple data.

USEFUL WEB RESOURCES

http://www.bbc.co.uk/schools/ks3bitesize/maths/
handling_data/index.shtml
http://www.gov.uk/government/publications/
public-spending-statistics

Chapter 18
. . . .
INTERPRETING DATA

LEARNING OUTCOMES

By the end of this chapter you should have a working knowledge of interpreting healthcare-related basic data.

As a healthcare professional, it is interesting to look at healthcare-related data. Viewing figures in health care comes in many different forms – maths in nursing is not all about working out how many tablets to give our patients!

SERIOUS HAZARDS OF TRANSFUSION

SHOT is the UK's haemovigilance scheme, standing for Serious Hazards of Transfusion. This organization collects and analyses adverse events and blood transfusion reactions in order to produce recommendations to improve patient safety in the transfusion process across the healthcare sector.

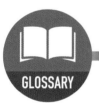

GLOSSARY

Haemovigilance

This is a set of surveillance procedures covering the entire blood transfusion chain, right from the donation and processing of blood and its components through to their provision and transfusion to patients, and their follow up.

Look at the chart below showing the summary of data for 2019. If I wanted to know how many patients receiving a blood transfusion experienced the adverse event of transfusion associated dyspnoea, I would first need to look at the key to find out the abbreviation for this. From this I can see that transfusion-associated dyspnoea is abbreviated as TAD. Then I look at the chart and see that 21 patients experienced this reaction. This does not mean that 21 patients in the UK in total actually experienced this reaction as I need to know the n number, which is shown to be 3397. Therefore, to get the actual number, I need to multiply 21 by 3397 = 71 337 patients.

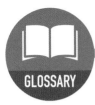

n = a variable representing a number, in this case 3397. This is the number of samples.

Serious Hazards of Transfusion
Summary of Data for 2019 N = 3397

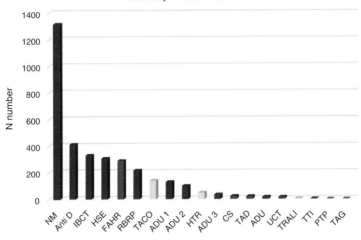

Source: Narayan,S. (ed). (2020). D. Polesetal et al. on behalf of the Serious Hazards of Transfusion (SHOT) Steering Group. The annual SHOT Report.

KEY POINTS

Summary data for 2019

N = 3397

NM	Near Miss 1314
Anti D	Anti D immunoglobulin 413
IBCT	Incorrect blood component transfused 329
HSE	Handling and storage errors 306

FAHR	Febrile, allergic and hypotensive reactions 288
RBRP	Right blood Right patient 216
TACO	Transfusion-associated circulatory overload 139
ADU 1	Delayed transfusion 129
ADU 2	Avoidable transfusion 99
HTR	Haemolytic transfusion reactions 49
ADU 3	Over or under transfusion 35
CS	Cell salvage 23
TAD	Transfusion-associated dyspnoea 21
ADU	Prothrombin complex concentrates (PCC) 16
UCT	Uncommon complications of transfusion 15
TRALI	Transfusion-related acute lung injury 3
TTI	Transfusion-transmitted infection 2
PTP	Post-transfusion purpura 0
TAGvHD	Transfusion-associated graft – vs-host disease 0

Red = Error
Blue = Not preventable
Yellow = Possibly preventable

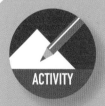

Activity 18.1

ACTIVITY

The bar chart above shows the Serious Hazards of (Blood) Transfusion audit showing the UK number of cases for the year 2019.

1 Where are the most hazards occurring?
2 What is the actual number of UK TRALI's?

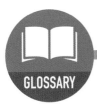

Dyspnoea

Dyspnoea means a difficulty breathing.

Post-transfusion Purpura

An adverse reaction to a blood transfusion causing a rash or redness.

Biochemistry Results

Blood glucose, sodium, potassium and other blood electrolytes are measured in millimoles or micromoles per litre of blood. This is how biochemistry results are presented.

A mole is the molecular weight of a substance in grams.

1 mole contains 1000 millimoles (mmol)

1 millimole contains 1000 micromoles (μmol)

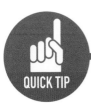

As a nurse you may see μ in laboratory test results: this means 'micro'. So, μmol means micromoles.

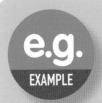

Let me show you an example. . .

A patient's laboratory results have just been returned. Patient A has a result of urea at 5.5 mmol/L. Let's look at Table 18.1 showing the safe ranges for blood electrolytes and other substances. The acceptable range for urea is 2.5–7.8 mmol/L, so this patient's urea is not a cause for concern.

Table 18.1 Biochemistry Results.

Test name	Units	Range Low	Range High
Sodium	mmol/L	133	146
Potassium	mmol/L	3.5	5.3
Urea	mmol/L	2.5	7.8
Chloride	mmol/L	95	108
Bicarbonate	mmol/L	22	26
Phosphate	mmol/L	0.8	1.5
Magnesium	mmol/L	0.7	1.0
Osmolality	mmol/kg	275	295
Alkaline phosphatase (ALP)	units, U/L	30	130
Creatine kinase (CK)	units, U/L	40 / 25	320 (M) / 200 (F)
Bilirubin (total)	μmol/L		<21
Adjusted calcium	mmol/L	2.2	2.6
Urate	μmol/L	200 / 140	430 (M) / 360 (F)
Carbamazepine	mg/L	4	12
Phenobarbitone	mg/L	10	40
Phenytoin	mg/L	5	20
Lithium	mmol/L	0.4	1.0
24 h urine urate	mmol/24 h	1.5	4.5
24 h urine phosphate	mmol/24 h	15	50
24 h urine magnesium	mmol/24 h	2.4	6.5

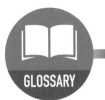

GLOSSARY

Normal bicarbonate level is 22–26 MEG = milliequivalents per litre of blood. A bicarbonate level above 26 is considered abnormally high and a level below 22 is considered abnormally low. Bicarbonate is a chemical buffer that keeps the pH of blood from ending up becoming too acidic.

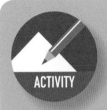

ACTIVITY

Activity 18.2

Patient B's results have just been returned. Here they are:

Sodium	145 mmol/L
Bicarbonate	30 mmol/L

Looking at the table, are these results within the acceptable range?

Arterial Blood Gas Testing

A common blood test performed in critical care areas is the arterial blood gas analysis, abbreviated to ABG's. Arterial blood is usually obtained from the wrist (radial artery). ABG's provide the following information: oxygenation, adequancy of ventilation and acid–base levels. Normal values can be seen in Figure i below

Figure i ABG Normal Values

PaO_2	This is oxygen	75–100 mmHg
$PaCO_2$	This is carbon dioxide	34–45 mmHg
pH	7.35–7.45	

Figure ii shows primary acid–base disturbances, in other words, what you would expect to see with these conditions:

Respiratory Acidosis Low pH. High PaCO$_2$. Normal or high normal Bicarbonate

Possible cause: intrinsic lung disease

Respiratory Alkalosis High pH. Low PaCO$_2$. Normal or high normal Bicarbonate

Possible cause: hyperventilation due to pain

Metabolic Acidosis Low pH. Normal or low normal PaCO$_2$. Low Bicarbonate

Possible cause: Accumulation of acid due to drugs

Metabolic Alkalosis High pH. Normal PaCO$_2$. High Bicarbonate

Possible Causes: Vomiting, burns

GLOSSARY

Respiratory acidosis occurs when the lungs can't remove enough of the carbon dioxide (CO$_2$) produced by the body. Excess CO$_2$ causes the pH of the blood to become too acidic.

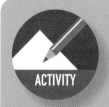

ACTIVITY

Activity 18.3

1 A patient has been vomiting +++. Results are: High pH, Normal PaCO$_2$. High Bicarbonate. What could these results indicate?

2 Patient B has been admitted to hospital due to an exacerbation of his asthma. Laboratory results show: Low pH. High PaCO$_2$. High normal Bicarbonate. What could these results indicate?

Covid 19

Covid-19 is a disease caused by an infection of the SARS-Cov-2 virus (a coronavirus) first identified in the city of Wuhan, in Chinas Hubei Province in December 2019. In March 2020, COVID-19 was declared a global pandemic.

Below Table 18.2 shows a snapshot of rates of new coronavirus infections per 100 000 people for districts in the West Country of England for the week up to 1 January 2021 and the week up to the 8th January 2021.

Table 18.2

Area	Week to 1 January 2021	Week to 8 January 2021
Bristol	376	503
Bath and North East Somerset	309	400
Cotswold	288	258
South Gloucestershire	383	455
Gloucester	496	491
Cheltenham	251	333
Dorset	281	354
Forest of Dean	400	449
Wiltshire	285	383
Swindon	528	552
Stroud	258	225
Tewkesbury	286	342
Mendip	265	278
South Somerset	265	285
North Somerset	360	390
Somerset West and Taunton	449	380
Sedgemoor	481	424

Source: Based on rates of new coronavirus. Public Health England, 2020/2021.

Activity 18.4

1 Which area had the largest number of cases per 100 000 for the week up to 1 January 2021?
2 Which area had the largest number of cases per 100 000 for the week up to 8 January 2021?
3 Which area had the lowest number of cases per 100 000 for the week up to 1 January 2021?
4 Which area had the lowest number of cases per 100 000 for the week up to 8 January 2021?
5 On the 8 January 2021, which areas had a reduction in numbers from the 1 January 2021 figures?
6 **a)** What is the mean average for infection rates for 1 January 2021?
  b) What is the mean average for infection rates for 8 January 2021?

Covid-19 Vaccinations

Below is some information about some of the Covid-19 vaccinations (Figure ii):

Figure ii

Name	Cost Per Dose	Storage	Number of Injections Required	Reported Efficiency of the Vaccines
Pfizer BioNTech	£14.80 per dose	Frozen: Minus 60 to minus 80 degrees Celsius	2	95%
Moderna	£24–£28 per dose	Frozen: Minus 15 to minus 25 degrees Celsius	2	94.5%
Oxford University/ AstraZeneca	£2.23 per dose	Fridge: 2 to 8 degrees Celsius	2	62–90%

These vaccines work by different modes, i.e., live vaccines, inactivated vaccines and genetically engineered vaccines, etc. When viewing these figures is it important to look at the whole picture, such as which vaccine is more cost-effective, how much are the hidden costs, such as the storage costs, and what are the reported efficiency rates of the vaccines, etc.

NOTE: The first trials for the Covid-19 vaccines did not include children.

Below are some of the global vaccine orders for three of the vaccines for Covid-19 (Figure iii):

Figure iii

European Union (EU)	Moderna Pfizer Oxford	160 million 300 million 400 million
USA	Moderna Pfizer Oxford	100 million 100 million 500 million
Canada	Moderna Pfizer Oxford	56 million 20 million 20 million
United Kingdom (UK)	Moderna Pfizer Oxford	15 million 40 million 100 million
Japan	Moderna Pfizer Oxford	50 million 120 million 120 million
Australia	Pfizer Oxford	10 million 33.8 million

Activity 18.5

1 How much will the financial bill be for 1 dose of the Oxford vaccine for:
   (a) the EU
   (b) the UK
2 How much will the financial bill for 1 dose of the Moderna vaccine, at £28 per dose, for:
   (a) Canada
   (b) Australia
3 How much will the financial bill be for 2 doses of the Pifzer vaccine for:
   (a) Japan
   (b) the UK
4 The Moderna vaccine comes in a multi-dose vial and contains enough vaccine for 10 doses. Each vaccine administered is 0.5 mLs. How much vaccine does the vial contain?

KEY POINTS

- Looking at biochemistry and arterial gases results.
- Looking at the moles, millimoles and micromoles.
- Looking at Public Health data and finances.

USEFUL WEB RESOURCES

http://www.bbc.co.uk/schools/ks3bitesize/maths/
   handling_data/index.shtml
Public Health England: https://coronavirus.data.gov.uk
SHOT: https://www.shotuk.org
World Health Organisation: https://www.who.int
https://covid19.who.int

Chapter 19

· · · · · · · · · · · · · · · · · · · ·

EMPLOYMENT SERVICES – SAMPLE TEST QUESTIONS

Calculation Skills for Nurses, Second Edition. Claire Boyd.
© 2022 John Wiley & Sons Ltd. Published 2022 by John Wiley & Sons Ltd.

Many healthcare employers now include a test of calculations competence at the interview stage. Talk about added pressure! You may wonder how I know what's in these test questions. Well, the simple answer to this is that I actually write many of them for my own NHS trust and others!

This chapter gives an example of sample questions in actual test papers for newly-qualified student nurses. Some employers allow calculators, but others may not, and pass rates are variable from trust to trust. For example, 60% may be the pass rate at one trust, 100% may be the pass rate at another. You may wish to gather your formula sheet for this exercise, as some trusts may include these at the start of the paper but, again, others may not.

There are other sample test questions for Nursing Associates, Assistant Practitioners, Paediatric Nurses, Mental Health Nurses, Learning Disabilities Nurses and Nurse Prescribers. Have a go at doing all the sample questions, no matter what your healthcare title, to build your maths competence.

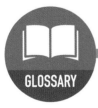

GLOSSARY

Pre-employment Calculations Test
A test used to determine competence in maths skills.

Now, let's see how you do in answering the questions in this sample test paper, Activity 19.1. You may not use a calculator. The activity is designed to assess your ability to calculate doses from a prescription. The process of calculating doses is the same regardless of the drug prescribed, or the age, clinical setting or diagnosis of the patient.

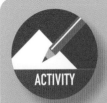

Activity 19.1

NOTE: you have 1 hour to complete this test.

1 Gentamicin is dispensed as 80 mg in 2 mL. The prescription is to administer 50 mg of gentamicin. What volume of gentamicin do you administer?

2 IV metronidazole 500 mg is dispensed in a 100 mL bag. A child is prescribed 300 g of metronidazole. What volume do you administer?

3 A patient is prescribed 60 mg of codeine phosphate. The drug is presented in tablets of 30 mg. How many tablets does the patient require?

4 Paracetamol is prescribed as 10 mg/kg and needs to be given 8 hourly. How much would you give to a baby weighing 2.5 kg?

5 1000 mL of sodium chloride 0.9% is prescribed to run over 12 hours. Calculate the drip rate in drops per minute.

6 Heparin is dispensed as 25 000 units in 5 mL. 30 000 units of heparin is prescribed, to be diluted to 48 mL.
   a. What volume of heparin would you administer?
   b. How much dilutant is required?

7 A woman has been prescribed 450 mL of blood, to run over 4 hours. Calculate the drip rate per minute using a filtered-blood administration set.

8 600 mL of fluid is dripping at 20 drops per minute. The IV set delivers 15 drops/mL. How long will the infusion take?

9 Hydrocortisone is dispensed as 100 mg in 2 mL. The patient is prescribed 75 mg of hydrocortisone. What volume of the drug would you administer?

10 A patient is prescribed 225 mg of ranitidine. Each tablet contains 150 mg. How many tablets does the patient require?

SAMPLE TEST QUESTIONS FOR NURSING ASSOCIATES

These are typical medication calculations test questions for Nursing Associates:

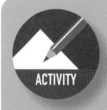

Activity 19.2

ACTIVITY

1 A doctor has prescribed patient A Risperidone 50 mg. Stock dose available is 25 mg/10 mL. What volume is required?

2 Patient B has been prescribed 40 mg ketamine. Stock dose available is 50 mg/5 mL. What volume is required?

3 Heparin has been prescribed for patient C as 20 000 units. Stock dose available is 4000 units/5 mL. What volume is required?

4 Stock dose of Tramadol is 50 mg/2 mL. Patient D has been prescribed 80 mg of Tramadol. What volume is required?

5 A patient is prescribed Budesonide 2000 micrograms by nebuliser. The medication is available as 300 micrograms/3 mL. What volume is required?

6 Prescribed: erythromycin
Stock: 300 mg in 10 mL
What volume do you draw up?

7 Prescribed: atropine 0.5 mg
Stock: 0.6 mg in 1 mL
What volume do you draw up?

8 Prescribed: heparin 1750 units
Stock: 1000 units/mL
What volume do you draw up?

9 Prescribed: Dexamethasone 3 mg
Stock: 4 mg/mL
What volume do you draw up?

10 Prescribed: Ranitidine 40 mg
Stock: 50 mg/2 mL
What volume do you draw up?

SAMPLE TEST QUESTIONS FOR ASSISTANT PRACTITIONERS

These are typical medication calculations test questions for Nursing Practitioners:

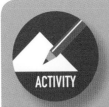

Activity 19.3

1   A patient is having an anaphylaxis episode and requires adrenaline urgently. Adrenaline is presented as 1 mg in 1 mL (1:1000). A nurse needs to administer 500 mcg IM now. How many mLs is this?

2   A woman has been prescribed a litre of 0.9% Sodium Chloride. The solution is to run over 5 hours. Calculate the drip rate in drops/min. The IV giving set delivers 20 drops/mL.

3   A patient has been prescribed 500 mg of oral paracetamol. Each tablet contains 500 mg. How many tablets are required?

4   A drug has been prescribed at 20 mg per kg per day to a 120 kg man. The drug is to be given 4 hourly. Calculate a single dose.

5   An insulin infusion containing 50 IU of Human Actrapid has been diluted with 50 mLs of sodium chloride, which has been running at:
    4.5 mLs/hr for 3 hours
    4.0 mLs/hr for 2 hours
    2 mLs/hr for 2 hours
    3.0 mLs/hr for 1 hour
    3.5 mLs/hr for 4 hours
    How many units of Actrapid insulin in total has the patient received?

6   Salbutamol nebuliser solutions for inhalation come in other size vials but presently in stock are only 2 mg/mL vials. Your patient has been prescribed 5.5 mg 4 times per day. How many mLs of the solution is required for a single dose?

7   A patient is to be given 1 litre of Sodium Chloride 0.9% over 10 hours. Calculate the drip rate in drops/min. The IV set delivers 20 drops/mL.

8   Not all healthcare environments have piped-in oxygen, instead relying on the oxygen being administered to patients via cylinders of varying capacity. This is also useful if the patient has to leave the bedside area to be transported to other departments and needs this continuous oxygen during transit. It is therefore useful for healthcare staff to work out how much oxygen is left in the cylinder so that the patient does not stop receiving this vital drug. Look at the chart below showing oxygen cylinder capacity.

Oxygen cylinder capacity					
Cylinder size Gas type Capacity(Litres)	CD Oxygen 460.0	E Oxygen 680.0	HX Oxygen 2300	G Oxygen 3400	J Oxygen 6800
Flow Rate (Litres)	Hours	Hours	Hours	Hours	Hours
1.00	7.7	11.3	38.3	56.7	113.3
2.00	3.8	5.7	19.2	28.3	56.7
3.00	2.6	3.8	12.8	18.9	37.8
4.00	1.9	2.8	9.6	14.2	28.3
5.00	1.5	2.3	7.7	11.3	22.7
6.00	1.3	1.9	6.4	9.4	18.9
7.00	1.1	1.6	5.5	8.1	16.2
8.00	1.0	1.4	4.8	7.1	14.2
9.00	0.9	1.3	4.3	6.3	12.6
10.00	0.8	1.1	3.8	5.7	11.3
11.00	0.7	1.0	3.5	5.2	10.3
12.00	0.6	0.9	3.2	4.7	9.4
13.00	0.6	0.9	2.9	4.4	8.7
14.00	0.5	0.8	2.7	4.0	8.1
15.00	0.5	0.8	2.6	3.8	7.6

Cylinder capacity (litres)/Flow rate (lpm)/60=hours supply

If a type J cylinder runs at 8 litres per minute, how many hours supply are there left?

NOTE: Formula = cylinder capacity (litres) divided by flow rate (litres per minute) divided by 60 = hours supply.

SAMPLE TEST QUESTIONS FOR PAEDIATRIC NURSES AND MIDWIVES

These are typical medication calculations test questions for Paediatric Nurses and Midwives:

Activity 19.4

1   A child requires Alfentanil. The Alfentanil is dispensed as 5 mg/mL. The prescription asks for the prescribed 2 mg to be diluted in 0.9% Sodium Chloride to give a total volume of 50 mLs. The child is to have 0.2 mg/hr.
   a.   How many mLs of Alfentanil do you draw up?
   b.   How many mLs of saline do you require to make the solution up to 50 mLs?
   c.   How many mLs/hr do you need to set the pump?
2   Paediatric IV Digoxin comes as 50 micrograms/2 mLs. The prescription is to administer 40 micrograms. What volume of Digoxin would you administer?
3   A baby weighing 2.2 kg is prescribed Vitamin K at 0.4 mg/kg IM. What dose should be prescribed and how is it given?
4   Benzylpenicillin IV is prescribed as 50 mg/kg. Baby weighs 4.2 kg.
   a.   What dose is prescribed?
   b.   It comes as 600 mg in 4 mls of water. How much do you give?
5   Vancomycin is prescribed at 15 mg/kg BD. Baby weighs 975 grams.
   a.   What is the prescribed dose?
      Vancomycin comes as 500 mg in 10 ml. 1 ml is taken out (50 mg) and diluted 10 times to give a concentration of 50 mg in 10 ml. It is then infused over 1 hour.
   b.   How much is going to be infused?

6 Cefotaxime IV is prescribed at 50 mg/kg BD. Baby weighs 650 grams.

    a. What amount is prescribed?

    b. Cefotaxime comes as 500 mg in 5 mLs of water. What amount do you give?

7 Metronidazole IV is prescribed at 7.5 mg/kg. Baby weighs 3.64 kg.

    a. How much is prescribed?

    b. It comes as 50 mg in 10 mls, how much is given?

8 Flucloxacillin IV is prescribed at 50 mg/kg. Baby weighs 4.5 kg.

    a. How much is prescribed?

    b. It comes as 250 mg in 5 mL in water. How much do you give?

9 A morphine dose is calculated as 2 mg/kg for a concentrated solution.

    a. A baby weighs 3.1 kg. How much morphine is prescribed?
Use this formula:
Amount in mgs (your answer from 9a) × by 1000 (to convert to mcg/kg/hour). Divide by 50 (mLs of fluid in the syringe), then divide by infant's weight, × by rate infusion is prescribed at:
Mg × 1000 ÷ 50 ÷ weight × rate = mcg per kg per hour

    b. The pump is running at 0.5 ml/hr. How many mcg/kg/hr is the baby receiving?

10 Dopamine is calculated as 120 mg/kg for a concentrated solution.

    a. Work out dose for the same baby (3.1 kg).
Use this formula:
Amount in mgs (your answer from 10a) × by 1000 (to convert to mcg/kg/hour).
Divide by 50 (mLs of fluid in the syringe), then divide by infant's weight, then divide by 60 to convert to per minute × by rate infusion is prescribed at:
Mg × 1000 ÷ 50 ÷ weight ÷ 60 × rate = mcg per kg per minute

    b. The pump is running at 0.25 mL/hr. How many mcg/kg/minute is the baby receiving?

SAMPLE TEST QUESTIONS FOR MENTAL HEALTH NURSES

These are typical calculations test questions for Mental Health Nurses:

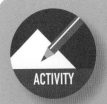

Activity 19.5

1 Patient A has been prescribed 6.5 mg Olanzapine IM injections for his schizophrenia and bipolar mania. Stock solution is 2.5 mg/mL. What volume do you administer?

2 Patient B has been prescribed 7.5 mg haloperidol per dose, to be administered three times per day for his Tourettes and schizophrenia. Stock ampoules come as 5 mg per 2 mL. What volume of the drug do you draw up?

3 Patient C has been prescribed 56 mg of transdermal selegiline, to be administered over a period of a week in equal amounts. Calculate the amount of drug to be administered per day.

4 A patient has been admitted to a mental health unit due to a mental health crisis. One of the drugs prescribed is ketamine 15 mg. Stock available is 50 mg/5 mL. What volume is required?

SAMPLE TEST QUESTIONS FOR LEARNING DISABILITIES NURSES

These are typical calculations test questions for Learning Disabilities Nurses:

Activity 19.6

1 A Service User has been prescribed Prednisolone 40 mg. The stock available is 5 mg/1 mL. What volume do you need to draw up to administer?

2 A Service User is prescribed Budesoride 1000 micrograms by nebuliser. Stock available is 500 microgram/1 mL ampoules. How many ampoules are required?

3 A Service User requires supplementary nutrition: 2500 mL Parenteral nutrition over 24 hours. Calculation the mL per hour the infusion pump should be set.

4 Work out this Service User's fluid balance:

INPUT	INPUT	OUTPUT
80 mL Tea	500 mL IV N/ Saline	150 mL Urine
100 mL Milk		200 mL Urine
50 mL Juice		70 mL Urine
200 mL Soup		250 mL Urine
70 mL Tea		
180 mL cocoa		500 mL Urine

Did you notice that all the test questions were quite similar, showing that all you need is a good solid mathematical base to work them all out.

NURSE PRESCRIBER SAMPLE TEST QUESTIONS

Nurses Prescribers need to go up a grade or two of maths competence and if you feel confident enough, have a go at their test questions. Do not use a calculator.

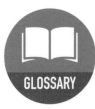

Nurse Prescriber

These are post graduate nurses who are licensed to issue medications to patients without a doctor being present or assessing the patient. Nurse Prescribers are also known as Non-Medical Prescribing Nurse (NMP), and are required to undertake post-graduate study.

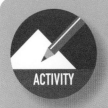

Activity 19.7

NMP Sample test questions

Maximum time is 30 minutes

100% Pass Rate

1   A drug is available as 2.5 milligram tablets. The dose is 7.5 milligrams daily for one week, followed by 10 milligrams daily for two weeks. How many tablets would you prescribe for this three weeks' supply?

2   A drug is available as 275 milligrams/3 millilitres intravenous injection. A patient requires 1 gram of the drug per dose. How many millilitres will you prescribe for each dose?

3   You need to prescribe a drug to a child weighing 11.5 kilograms. Your patient needs 100 mg/kilogram/day of this drug in two divided doses. How much of the drug will you need to prescribe per dose?

4   Drug X is available as 50 microgram tablets. The dose is 0.025 milligrams once a day. How many tablets would you need to prescribe for 14 days?

5   The dose of medicine for a child is 100 micrograms/kilogram body weight/day. Calculate the total daily dose needed in milligrams for a child weighing 28 kilograms?

KEY POINT

- Look at how to answer pre-employment test papers correctly.

USEFUL WEB RESOURCES

www.testandcalc.com/quiz/index.asp
www.nmc.org.uk

Chapter 20
BODY MASS INDEX

Calculation Skills for Nurses, Second Edition. Claire Boyd.

LEARNING OUTCOMES

By the end of this chapter you will have the knowledge to work out a patient's body mass index (BMI) and percentage weight loss.

Many care homes and institutions use the Malnutrition Universal Screening Tool (MUST) to identify malnourished or obese adult patients/service users, and the body mass index (BMI) chart is part of this assessment tool. Although we looked at this in Chapter 13, we still need to know what a body mass index means and how to obtain this figure. The MUST is shown in Appendix 2.

BODY MASS INDEX

The Body Mass Index (BMI) is a measurement that uses your height and weight to work out if your weight is healthy. This has been particularly important to assess during the Coronavirus pandemic, as individuals who are overweight have been deemed to be at higher risk. The BMI calculator divides weight in kilograms by their height in metres squared.

$$\text{BMI} = \text{weight}\left(\text{kg}\right) / \text{height}\left(\text{m}^2\right)$$

Let me show you an example:

If a patient weighs 74 kg and is 1.74 metres tall, the BMI can be calculated by first working out the height in metres squared = 1.74 × 1.74 = 3.0276, and then dividing the weight of 74 kg by this number.

$$BMI = \frac{Weight}{HEIGHT \ (M^2)} \quad \frac{74}{1.74 \times 1.74}$$

$$= \frac{74}{3.0276} = 24.4 \ kg/m^2$$

Activity 20.1

What is the above patient's weight status on the BMI chart in Figure i below?

Fig i

BMI	Weight Status
Below 18.5	Underweight
18.5–24.9	Normal/Healthy
25–29.9	Overweight
30–39.9	Obese
Above 40	Very obese

Although the BMI does compare well with body fatness for most people, it is not a definite indicator of a percentage of an individual's body fat. The correlation between body fat and BMI also has some variables:

- Women tend to have more body fat than men at the same BMI.
- Older people, on average, tend to have more body fat than younger adults at the same BMI
- Athletes have a high BMI due to their increased muscularity rather than increased body fatness

Activity 20.2

Work out the BMI of the following patients and their weight status:

Height	Weight
1 1.75 metres	93.5 kg
2 1.67 metres	79 kg
3 1.84 metres	47.2 kg
4 1.57 metres	72.6 kg
5 1.54 metres	80 kg
6 1.82 metres	62 kg
7 1.61 metres	88 kg
8 1.86 metres	78 kg
9 1.66 metres	65 kg
10 1.86 metres	79 kg

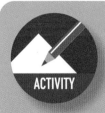

Activity 20.3

Patient A weighs 105 kg and is 1.65 m in height. Using the steps above, find out the patient's BMI and round up your answer.

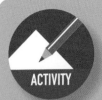

Activity 20.4

Find out your height in metres and your weight in kilograms. Then, using the steps above, find out **your** BMI.

WEIGHT LOSS

Weight can be variable – we don't just put on weight, but can lose it as well. To work out weight loss as a percentage, you can use this formula:

$$\text{Percentage weight loss} = \frac{(\text{Usual weight kg} - \text{Actual weight kg})}{\text{Usual weight kg}} \times 100$$

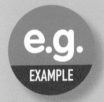

Maria Groban is admitted to a Nursing Home weighing 59 kg. Three months later her weight has fallen to 54 kg. Using the formula to work out the percentage weight loss:

Usual weight 59 kg

Actual weight now 54 kg

$$\frac{59\text{kg} - 54\text{kg}}{59\text{kg} \times 100} = 8.47$$

If you don't want to use a calculator, you can break this down into bite-size chunks:

1 $59 - 54 = 5$
2 $5/59 = 0.084$
3 To get the percentage amount: $0.084 \times 100 = 8.47$

Therefore, Maria has lost 8.47, approximately 8.5% of her body weight.

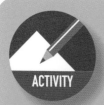

ACTIVITY

Activity 20.5

Ernest Taylor was admitted to hospital weighing 79 kg. Two months later, this has fallen to 75 kg. What is Ernest's percentage weight lost?

Usual weight 79 kg

Actual weight now 75 kg

KEY POINT

- How to work out an adult's body mass index and weight loss as a percentage.

USEFUL WEB RESOURCES

https://www.nhs.uk/live-well/healthy-weight/bmi-calculator

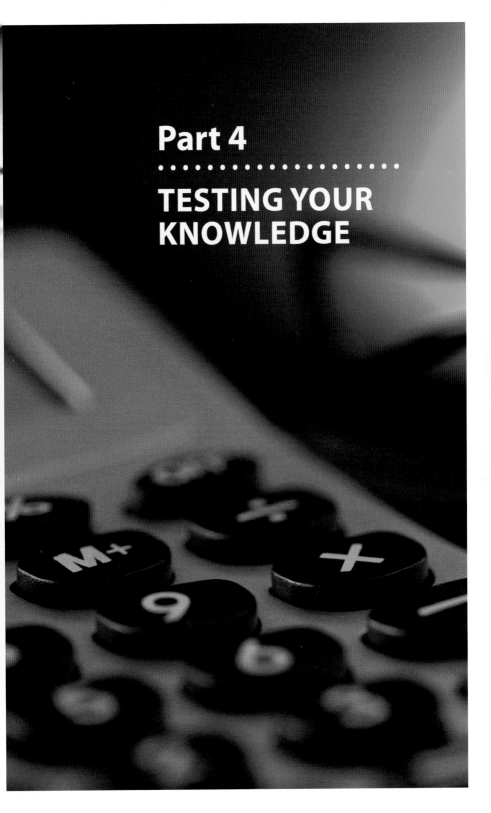

Part 4

. . . .

TESTING YOUR KNOWLEDGE

Chapter 21

. . . .

KNOWLEDGE TESTS

Calculation Skills for Nurses, Second Edition. Claire Boyd.
© 2022 John Wiley & Sons Ltd. Published 2022 by John Wiley & Sons Ltd.

These knowledge tests have been compiled to test your knowledge of everything we have looked at throughout the book, and to show you the calculation problems you may come across in your healthcare career. Perhaps you don't feel quite ready to work through one of these knowledge tests at the moment so let's work through one together. I have done the working out for you so you just need to add the actual answer. Or, if you prefer, just ignore the middle column of the below:

QUESTION	WORKING OUT	ANSWER
1 Convert 7.8 kg to grams	Larger unit kg to smaller unit g = × 1000 7.8 × 1000 =	
2 Convert 7555 mcg to mg	Smaller unit mcg to larger unit mg = /1000 7555/1000 =	
3 Convert 1.7 litres to mL	Larger unit l to smaller unit mL = × 1000 1.7 × 1000 =	
4 Convert 43 mL to litres	Smaller unit mL to larger unit l = /1000 43/1000 =	
5 Convert 3.56 g to mg	Larger unit g to smaller unit mg = × 1000 3.56 × 1000 =	
6 Convert 25 mcg to mg	Smaller unit mcg to larger unit mg = /1000 25/000 =	
7 Convert 777 mg to grams	Smaller unit mg to larger unit g = /1000 777/1000 =	
8 Convert 0.5 litres to mL	Larger unit l to smaller unit mL = × 1000 0.5 × 1000 =	
9 Convert 451 mL to litres	Smaller unit mL to larger unit l = /1000 451/1000 =	
10 Convert 1.9 metres to centimetres	Larger unit m to smaller unit cm = 1.9 × 1000 =	

QUESTION	WORKING OUT	ANSWER
11 A patient has been prescribed 300 mg of a drug every 4 hours. The stock tablets on hand are 150 mg. How many tablets do you need to give to the patient in a day?	24 Hours 4 Hourly = Means that the drug needs to be administered 6 times per day. 300 mg (prescribed dose) × 6 = 1800 mg per day. $\dfrac{WYW}{WYG} = \dfrac{1800\ mg}{150\ mg} =$ Don't forget to divide your answer by 6, as tablets to be administered every 4 hours	
12 A drug error has been made. 0.1 mL of a drug has been administered to a patient when it should have been 0.01 mL. How many times too much is this?	This is a factor of 10, meaning the decimal point on 0.1 should have been moved once to the left. Or, 0.1/10 = 0.01 mL =	
13 A patient requires 500 mcg of a drug. You have an ampoule of the drug presented as 1 mg in 1 mL. How many mLs do you give?	First convert the 500 mcg into mg = 500/1000 = 0.5 mg. then use formula = $\dfrac{WYW}{WYG \times VOL}\ \dfrac{0.5\ mg}{1.0\ mg \times 1\ mL} =$	
14 35 units of insulin has been prescribed. It is dispensed as 100 units in 1 mL. How many mLs do you administer?	$\dfrac{WYW}{WYG \times VOL}\ \dfrac{35\ units}{100\ units \times 1} =$	

QUESTION	WORKING OUT	ANSWER
15 A patient is given 2 litres of 0.45% saline. How many grams of sodium will the patient receive?	Change 2 litres into mL = 2 l = 2000 mLs. $\dfrac{2000 \times 0.45}{100} =$	
16 A patient weighs 60 kg and requires 40 mcg/kg of a drug. **A** How many mcg are required? **B** How many mg is this?	**(a)** Weight × Dose = 60 kg × 40 mcg = **(b)** Change mcg into mg = 2400/1000 =	
17 How many grams of medication do you have in 15g of 12% w/w ointment?	$\dfrac{15 \times . 12}{100} =$	
18 A patient has been prescribed ibuprofen 5 mg/mg/dose. She weighs 65 kg. Calculate how much ibuprofen you need to administer.	Weight × dose 65 kg × 5 mg =	
19 A patient has been prescribed 20 mL of lactulose b.d. How many full days' supply of lactulose is there in a 500 mL bottle?	First remember b.d = twice a day, therefore patient requires 40 mLs of lactulose per day. How many lots of 40 mLs can I get out of a 500 mL bottle?	

QUESTION	WORKING OUT	ANSWER
20 A patient is prescribed 9 mg of morphine. Stock solution is 15 mg in 1 mL. How much do you administer?	$\dfrac{WYW}{WYG \times VOL}$ $\dfrac{9\ mg}{15\ mg \times 1\ mL} =$	

Now get comfortable, sharpen those pencils and let's begin the big boy knowledge tests!

KNOWLEDGE TEST 1

1 Waterlow Pressure Ulcer Prevention/Treatment: Walter Jones is an 80-year-old male with a BMI of 20 kg/m². Walter has oedematous legs and has Type 2 diabetes. Walter has a good appetite. Presently, he has been restricted in his mobility due to his swollen legs. What is Walter's Waterlow score?

2 National Early Warning Score (NEWS 2): Jane Fielding has the following observations:

Respiratory rate Scale 1	18 breaths per minute
SpO_2	99% Air
Blood pressure	130/80
Heart rate	80 bpm
Neurological response	Alert
Temp	37.1 degrees Celsius

What is her NEWS score?

3 A patient has been prescribed 35 mg of codeine phosphate by injection. Ampoules of 60 mg in 1 mL are available. How many millilitres will you administer?

4 A patient is prescribed 27 mg of Adenocor. Stock ampoules contain 30 mg in 10 mL. What volume of drug needs to be administered?

5 A drug is presented as 4 g in 400 mL. A patient weighing 100 kg is prescribed 10 mg/kg/h of the drug.

(a) How many milligrams per hour of the drug does the patient need?

(b) How many millilitres per hour do you set the infusion pump at?

6 Furosemide is available in a concentration of 20 mg in 2 mL. A patient is prescribed 15 mg intravenously as a bolus. It is to be given at a maximum rate of 3 mg/minute.

(a) What volume of furosemide would you administer?

(b) How many minutes should it be given over?

7 IV morphine sulphate comes as 15 mg in 1 mL. The prescription is to administer 6 mg of morphine sulphate. What volume of the drug would you administer?

8 Amoxicillin is presented as 500 mg per ampoule. It is to be diluted to a volume of 10 mL. Your patient is prescribed 1.5 g. What volume of amoxicillin do you draw up?

9 Caffeine base is prescribed at 2.5 mg/kg per 24 hours. The patient, a baby, weighs 1.2 kg.

(a) What amount of caffeine base is prescribed?

(b) Caffeine base comes as 5 mg in 1 mL. This needs to be reconstituted five times with 0.9% sodium chloride (NaCl) and infused over 10 minutes.

What is the total volume to be infused?

10 Benzylpenicillin IV is prescribed to a baby as 50 mg/kg. The baby weighs 3.4 kg.

(a) What dose is prescribed?

(b) The drug comes as 600 mg in 4 mL of water. How much do you give?

KNOWLEDGE TEST 2

1 Malnutrition Universal Screening Tool (MUST): Max Norman is a 52-year-old male. He is 5 feet 8½ inches in height and weighs 100 kg. What is his BMI?

2 National Early Warning Score (NEWS 2): Robert Hayes
   has the following observations:

Respiratory rate	36 breaths per minute
SpO$_2$	89% on air
Scale 1	
Blood pressure	108/70 mmHg
Heart rate	129 beats per minute
Neurological response	Alert
Temp:	38.4 Degrees Celsius

   What is his NEWS score?

3 A patient has been prescribed 75 mg of pethidine by
   injection. 50 mg in 1 mL of liquid for injection is
   available. How many millilitres will you administer?

4 A patient is prescribed 75 micrograms of fenatyl citrate
   intravenously. 0.1 mg in 1 mL of liquid for IV injection is
   available. How many millilitres will you administer?

5 Digoxin ampoules contain 500 micrograms in 2 mL.
   What volume is needed for an injection of
   275 micrograms?

6 Ampoules of adrenaline for anaphylactic shock contain
   1 mg in 1 mL (1,1000). What volume is needed for an
   IM injection of 500 micrograms?

7 Ampicillin 80 mg/kg per day is prescribed for a
   90 kg man. The drug is to be given 6 hourly.
   Calculate the amount needed for a single dose.

8 Benzylpenicillin IV is prescribed as 50 mg/kg. The
   patient, a baby, weighs 4.2 kg.
   (a) What dose is prescribed?
   (b) The drug comes as 600 mg in 4 mL of water. How
       much do you give?

9 A patient is to have 2 L of clear fluids in 24 hours. He
   has received 700 mL in 10 hours. How many drops per
   minute are required to correct the infusion?

10 An insulin infusion containing 50 units of human
   Actrapid has been diluted with 50 mL of sodium
   chloride, which has been running at:

3 mL / hour for 1 hour
3.5 mL / hour for 2 hours
2 mL / hour for 2 hours
2.5 mL / hour for 2 hours
4 mL / hour for 1 hour

How many units of Actrapid insulin in total has the patient received?

KNOWLEDGE TEST 3

1 Waterlow Pressure Ulcer Prevention/Treatment: Violet Simms is a 90-year-old lady with a BMI of 18 kg/m². Violet is covered in bruises due to falls, and has 'tissue paper' skin. Violet has gone off her food lately and is eating very poorly, causing her to lose approximately 1.8 kg in the last few weeks. Violet has been experiencing some urinary incontinence recently and has just been found to be suffering from a high temperature. Violet is reluctant to mobilise independently since her falls and now uses a wheelchair during the day. What is Violet's Waterlow score?

2 National Early Warning Score (NEWS 2): Simon Patrick has the following observations:

Respiratory rate Scale 1	20 breaths per minute
SpO$_2$	96% on air
Blood pressure	120/71 mmHg
Heart rate	100 beats per minute
Neurological response	Alert
Temp	38.0 Degrees Celsius
What is his NEWS 2 score?	

3 A patient is prescribed 22 mg of gentamicin by injection. 20 mg in 2 mL of liquid for IM injection is available. How many millilitres will you administer?

4 A patient has been prescribed 30 mg of furosemide intravenously. 20 mg in 2 mL of liquid for IV injection is available. How many millilitres do you administer?

5 Diamorphine hydrochloride 10 mg is to be reconstituted in 10 mL of water for injection. A patient is prescribed a 20 mg bolus intramuscular injection. What volume of the drug needs to be administered?
NOTE: there is no displacement value to be considered.

6 Atenolol is available in a concentration of 5 mg in 10 mL. The patient is prescribed 2.5 mg IV as a bolus. It is to be given at a maximum rate of 1 mg/minute.
(a) What volume of atenolol would you administer?
(b) How many minutes should it be given over?

7 A patient is to receive 3 mg/mL of Adenocor, followed by a further 6 mg, then 12 mg, over a period of 6 minutes. What volume does the patient receive in total?

8 A morphine dose is calculated as 2 mg/kg for a concentrated solution.
(a) A baby weighs 3.1 kg: how much morphine is prescribed for this infant?
(b) The pump is running at 0.5 mL/hour. How many micrograms/kg per hour is the baby receiving?

9 500 mL of fluid is dripping at 35 drops per minute. The IV set delivers 15 drops/mL. How long will the infusion take?

10 Dopamine 150 mg is added to a bag of 500 mL of 5% dextrose. The prescription is to administer 6 micrograms/kg per minute of the infusate to a 75 kg patient. At what rate (in mL/hour) do you set the infusion pump?

KNOWLEDGE TEST 4

1 Malnutrition Universal Screening Tool (MUST): Sarah Hann is a 92-year-old lady who is 5 feet 4 inches in height and weighs 44 kg. What is her BMI?

2 National Early Warning Score (NEWS 2): Lesley David has the following observations:

Respiratory rate	10 breaths per minute
Scale 2	
SpO$_2$	90% on air
Blood pressure	99/60 mmHg
Heart rate	51 beats per minute
Neurological response	Newly confused
Temp	37 Degrees Celsius
What is his NEWS 2 score?	

3 A patient has been prescribed 200 mg of coamoxiclav. 600 mg in 10 mL of liquid for IV injection is available. How many millilitres do you administer?

4 Vancomycin is presented as a 1 g ampoule. It is to be diluted in 20 mL of water for injection. Your patient is prescribed 500 mg.

  (a) What volume of vancomycin do you draw up? The vancomycin is to be added to a 500 mL bag of 0.9% saline. It is to be given at a rate of 4 mg/minute, due to the patient's fluid restriction.

  (b) How many minutes must the infusion be given over?

  (c) You are going to run it through an infusion pump. At what rate (in mL/hour) would you set the infusion pump?

5 A woman has been prescribed one unit of blood. The transfusion is to run over 3 hours. The unit consists of 350 mL of blood. The IV giving set (filtered) delivers 15 drops/mL. Calculate the drip rate in drops per minute.

6 Diamorphine hydrochloride 10 mg is to be reconstituted in 10 mL of water for injection. A patient is prescribed a 5 mg bolus intramuscular injection. What volume of the drug needs to be administered?

7 1000 mL of fluid is dripping at 20 drops per minute. The IV set delivers 15 drops/mL. How long will the infusion take?

8 Vancomycin is prescribed at 15 mg/kg BD. A baby patient weighs 975 g.

    (a) What is the prescribed dose? Vancomycin comes as 500 mg in 10 mL. 1 mL is taken out (50 mg) and diluted 10 times to give a concentration of 50 mg in 10 mL. It is then infused over 1 hour.

    (b) How much is going to be infused?

9 A patient weighing 65 kg is prescribed 500 micrograms/kg/h of aminophylline. 250 g of aminophylline has been added to 100 mL of fluid.

    (a) How many mg/hour of aminophylline does the patient require?

    (b) At what rate (in millilitres per hour) would you set the infusion pump?

10 A patient weighing 70 kg has been prescribed 1.5 mg/kg of enoxaparin post-surgery. What amount do you administer?

USEFUL WEB RESOURCES

www.testandcalc.com/quiz/index.asp
http://www.bnf.org/bnf/bnf/current/104945.htm

You will need to register to access the bnf site (but registration is free)

Answers to Activity Questions

Activity 1.1

1 11.6
2 92
3 43.85
4 3.2

If you got any of questions **1–4** wrong, why not take a look at Chapter 2. Don't worry, we all make mistakes. Keep calm and carry on!

5 0.8
6 0.3
7 4.7
8 2.3
9 9.5
10 3.4
11 2.42
12 9.23
13 0.92
14 0.52
15 2.34
16 6.71
17 0.826
18 1.587
19 39
20 32

21 40

If you got any of questions **5–21** wrong, why not take a look at the Decimals section in Chapter 2.

22 6 g
23 0.0007 mg
24 9000 ng
25 30 mg
26 2500 mL
27 92 000 g
28 8000 g
29 0.0645 mg
30 1.527 mg
31 0.00002 g
32 1200 micrograms

If you got any of the questions **22–32** wrong, why not take a look at the Metric Measures section in Chapter 2

33 125 mL
34 61.3%
35 23.3%

If you got questions **33–35** wrong, why not take a look at the Percentages section in Chapter 2.

36 0.8
37 35.0

Calculation Skills for Nurses, Second Edition. Claire Boyd.
© 2022 John Wiley & Sons Ltd. Published 2022 by John Wiley & Sons Ltd.

38 0.1

If you got any of questions **36–38** wrong, why not take a look at the Fractions section in Chapter 2.

39 1 in 5 = 1/5; 1/5 × 200 mL = 40 mL

40 1:5 = 1 in 6 = 1/6; 1/6 × 200 mL = 33 mL to the nearest millilitre

41 1/3 × 600 mL = 200 mL

If you got any of questions **39–41** wrong, why not take a look at the Ratios section in Chapter 2.

42 6/10 or 3/5

43 75%

44 $\dfrac{90}{180 \times 100} = 50\%$

If you got any of questions **42–44** wrong, why not take a look at the Percentages section in Chapter 2.

45 6.35 kg

46 1.35 kg

47 176.0 lbs

If you got any of questions **45–47** wrong, why not take a look at the Imperial weights section in Chapter 3.

48 19

49 4

50 60.48

If you got any of questions **48–50** wrong, why not take a look at the Averages section in Chapter 2.

Activity 2.1

135 grams – 18 grams = 117 mL

Activity 2.2

1 500 mg/25 = 20 mg/mL

2 20 mg/4 = 5 mg/mL

3 1000 mg/20 = 50 mg/mL

Activity 2.3

SECTION ONE

1 2.7

2 1.3

3 1.8

4 2.0

5 4.6

SECTION TWO

1 56

2 43

3 100

4 33

5 67

Activity 2.4

1 450/100 × 20 = 90 mL

2 1200/100 × 15 = 180 mL

3 240/300 × 100 = 80%

4 85/400 × 100 = 21.25%

Activity 2.5

1 8.3

2 7.5

3 35

4 20.8

5 41.7

6 17.4

Activity 2.6

a 1 gram in 1000 mL = 1000 mg in 1000 mL

$\dfrac{1000\ mg}{1000\ mL} = 1 mg$ per 1 mL

1 gram in 10 000 = 1000 mg in 10 000 mL

$\dfrac{1000\ mg}{10\ 000\ mL} = 0.1$ mg/mL (or 1 mg in 10 mL)

b The 1 in 10 000 solution is the weakest.

Activity 2.7

1 (i) 25 mL; (ii) 20 mL
2 (i) 566 mL; (ii) 500 mL
3 (i) 55 mL; (ii) 50 mL
4 (i) 200 mL; (ii) 150 mL

Activity 2.8

1 19 + 19 + 19.5 + 18.0 + 17 = 92.5/5 = 18.5 mmHg

Activity 3.1

SECTION ONE

1 6 g
2 39 L
3 0.35 L
4 0.00007 mg
5 4 kg
6 4.5 g
7 800 micrograms
8 9000 ng
9 1.3 kg
10 0.000462 g

SECTION TWO

1 720 mg
2 1400 micrograms
3 30 mg
4 0.002 kg
5 2500 mL
6 700 micrograms
7 61 250 mL
8 92 000 g
9 20 micrograms
10 0.000023 g

SECTION THREE

1 0.02 mg
2 0.634 kg
3 63.5 micrograms
4 250 ng
5 8000 g
6 1.527 mg
7 21 900 mL
8 0.0645 mg
9 0.3498 kg
10 0.05 L

SECTION FOUR

1 3000 mL
2 1200 micrograms
3 40 micrograms
4 120 mg
5 0.00002 g
6 20 ng
7 2386 g
8 0.004 micrograms
9 1.234 L
10 0.32 g

Activity 3.2

1 3
2 38
3 0.25
4 0.00005
5 2
6 2.5
7 300
8 6000
9 1.6
10 0.000375
11 95.25 + 4.5 = 99.75
12 13 stone (82.55 kg/6.35 kg)
13 400 micrograms = 0.4 mg; therefore, the patient has taken 0.8 mg.
14 75 micrograms
15 0.935 kilograms
16 0.125 mg
17 1400 mL

18 0.027 grams
19 750 mg
20 7000 picograms

Activity 3.3

1 97.5 cm
2 127 cm
3 32.5 cm
4 108 cm
5 61.7 cm
6 1130 mm
7 1020 mm
8 770 mm
9 981 mm
10 1900 mm

Activity 4.1a

1 2 tablets
2 ½ tablet
3 1½ tablets
4 The small amount needs to be converted into milligrams, which will result in an even smaller amount. To change micrograms into milligrams, divide by 1000 (going up to the next decimal unit), giving 0.5 micrograms = 0.0005 mg. Then:

$\dfrac{0.0005}{250} = 0.000002$ mg. This is not achievable but if this is the number you came up with then you are correct.

5 ½ tablet
6 1½ tablets

Activity 4.1b

1 62.5 + 62.5 = 125.0 = 2 tablets
2 5 mg + 2 mg + 2 mg = 9 mg = 3 tablets
3 $\dfrac{300}{200} = 1.5 = 1$½ tablets

4 160 mg + 160 mg = 320 mg = 2 tablets
5 50 mg + 25 mg = 75 mg = 2 tablets
6 $\dfrac{250}{100} = 2.5 = 2$½ tablets

Activity 4.2

a 65 × 25 – 1625 mg TDD
b A single dose = 1625/4 = 406.25 mg

Activity 5.1

1 $\dfrac{50\,mg}{80\,mg} \times 2\,mL = 1.25\,mL$
2 $\dfrac{400\,mg}{500\,mg} \times 100\,mL = 80\,mL$
3 $\dfrac{20\,000\,units}{25\,000\,units} \times 1\,mL = 0.8\,mL$
4 $\dfrac{600\,mg}{400\,mg} \times 3\,mL = 4.5\,mL$
5 500 micrograms = 0.5 mg/0.5 mL + 500 micrograms = 0.5 mg/0.5 mL = 1 mg in 1 mL
6 $\dfrac{30\,mg}{20\,mg} \times 5\,mL = 7.5\,mL$
7 Change 1.2 grams into milligrams = 1200 mg
$\dfrac{800\,mg}{1200\,mg} \times 6\,mL = 3.9\,mL$
8 $\dfrac{250\,mg}{125\,mg} \times 5\,mL = 10\,mL$
9 $\dfrac{0.5\,mg}{0.6\,mg} \times 1\,mL = 0.83\,mL$
10 $\dfrac{1750\,units}{1000\,units} \times 1\,mL = 1.75\,mL$

Activity 6.1

1

2

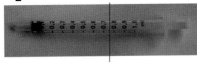

3 1.2 mL

Activity 6.2

Meniscus: approximately 29.0 mL

Activity 7.1

1 4 mL – 0.4 mL = 3.6 mL of water
2 Displacement value = 0.8 mL/1 g;
10 mL – 0.8 mL = 9.2 mL
3 Displacement value = 0.5 mL for
1 gram; 4 mL – 0.5 mL = 3.5 mL
4 Displacement value = 0.2 mL for
250 mg; 5 mL – 0.2 mL = 4.8 mL

Activity 8.1

1 Wrong: 15.5 kg × 8 mg = 124 mg
2 Wrong: 82.55 kg × 12 mg =
990.6 mg
3 Correct: 60 kg × 7.5 mg = 450 mg
4 Wrong: 42.9 kg × 10 mg = 429 mg
5 Wrong: 14.6 kg × .5 mg = 36 .5 mg
6 Correct: 88.9 kg × 8 mg =
711.2 mg
This prescriber needs to practice
his/her maths!

Activity 8.2

1 70 kg × 10 mg = 700 mg
2 2.5 kg × 10 mg = 25 mg daily.
Divide this by 3 (to get 8-hourly
doses) = 8.33 mg, three times a
day.
3 0.570 kg × 2 mg = 1.14 mg/day

4 148 kg × 30 mg = 1440 mg daily;
1440/3 = 480 mg/dose
5 15 kg × 40 mg = 600 mg daily;
600/4 = 150 mg/dose
6 20 kg × 80 mg = 1600 mg daily;
1600/4 = 400 mg/dose
7 58 kg × 100 mg = 5800 mg daily;
5800/4 = 1450 mg/dose
8 92 kg × 60 mg = 5520 mg daily;
5520/4 = 1380 mg/dose
9 35 kg × 20 mg = 700 mg daily;
700/3 = 233 mg/dose
10 20 kg × 45 mg = 900 mg daily;
900/4 = 225 mg/dose

Activity 9.1

1 500/2 = 250 mL/hr
2 2000/8 = 250 mL/hr
3 110/0.5 = 220 mL/hr
4 1000/2 = 500 mL/hr

Activity 9.2

1 First change 1.5 L into millilitres =
1500 mL
$$\frac{1500}{12} \times \frac{20}{60} = 41.66 = 42 \text{ drops per}$$
minute (nearest whole drop).
2 $\frac{420}{4} \times \frac{15}{60} = 26.25 = 26$ drops

per minutes

3 $\frac{150}{6} \times \frac{60}{60} = 25$ drops per minute

4 $\frac{350}{3} \times \frac{15}{60} = 29$ drops per minute

5 $\frac{500}{6} \times \frac{20}{60} = 27.77 = 28$ drops

per minutes

6 (25 × 24 = 600) + (30 × 24 = 720)
= 1320 mL in 24 hours

7 $\dfrac{1000}{6} \times \dfrac{20}{60} = 55.55 = 56\,\text{drops}$
per minutes

8 $\dfrac{1500}{10} \times \dfrac{20}{60} = 50\,\text{drops per minute}$

9 $\dfrac{260}{2} \times \dfrac{15}{60} = 32.5 = 33\,\text{drops}$
per minutes

10 $\dfrac{125}{1} \times \dfrac{15}{60} = 31.25 = 31\,\text{drops}$
per minutes

11 $\dfrac{200}{2} \times \dfrac{60}{60} = 100\,\text{drops per minute}$

12 $\dfrac{150}{4} \times \dfrac{60}{60} = 37.5 = 38\,\text{drops}$
per minutes

Activity 9.3

1 Fluid left to infuse: 3000 mL −
1500 mL = 1500 mL; hours left to
infuse: 24 − 8 = 16 hours
$\dfrac{1500}{16} \times \dfrac{20}{60} = 31.25 = 31\,\text{drops}$
per minute

2 $\dfrac{600}{20} \times \dfrac{15}{60} = 7.5 = 7\tfrac{1}{2}\,\text{hours}$

3 $\dfrac{1000}{20} \times \dfrac{15}{60} = 12.5 = 12\tfrac{1}{2}\,\text{hours}$

4 Fluid left to infuse: 2000 mL −
1500 mL = 500 mL; hours left to
infuse: 24 − 6 = 18 hours
$\dfrac{500}{18} \times \dfrac{20}{60} = 9.26 = 9\,\text{drops}$
per minute

5 $\dfrac{1000}{43} \times \dfrac{20}{60} = 7\tfrac{3}{4}\,\text{hours}$

Activity 10.1

1 $\dfrac{48\,\text{mL}}{24\,\text{hours}} = 2\,\text{mL / hour}$

2 3 mL × 2 hours = 6.0 mL
3.5 mL × 3 hours = 10.5 mL
2 mL × 1 hour = 2.0 mL
2.5 mL × 1 hour = 2.5 mL
4 mL × 2 hours = 8.0 mL
29.0 units of Actrapid have been
received in total.

3 $\dfrac{1000\,\text{mL}}{8\,\text{hours}} = 125\,\text{mL / hour}$

4 $\dfrac{500\,\text{mL}}{6\,\text{hours}} = 83.3\,\text{mL / hour}$

5 $\dfrac{48\,\text{mL}}{12\,\text{hours}} = 4\,\text{mL / hour}$

6 $\dfrac{1000\,\text{mL}}{12\,\text{hours}} = 83.3\,\text{mL / hour}$

7 $\dfrac{24\,\text{mL}}{12\,\text{hours}} = 2\,\text{mL / hour}$

8 $\dfrac{100\,\text{mL}}{0.5\,\text{hours}} = 200\,\text{mL / hour}$
(remember : 30 mins = 0.5 hours)

9 $\dfrac{80\,\text{mL}}{0.5\,\text{hours}} = 160\,\text{mL / hour}$

10 $\dfrac{75\,\text{mL} \times 60\,\text{minutes}}{20\,\text{minutes}} = 225\,\text{mL / hour}$
(remember to convert the 75 mL
per minute into an hourly rate).

Activity 10.2

1 $\dfrac{50\,\text{mL} \times 60\,\text{minutes}}{20\,\text{minutes}}$
$= 150\,\text{mL / hour}$

2 $\dfrac{100\,\text{mL} \times 60\,\text{minutes}}{30\,\text{minutes}}$
$= 200\,\text{mL / hour}$

3 $\dfrac{100\,\text{mL} \times 60\,\text{minutes}}{30\,\text{minutes}}$

$= 200\,\text{mL} / \text{hour}$

4 $\dfrac{120\,\text{mL} \times 60\,\text{minutes}}{50\,\text{minutes}}$

$= 144\,\text{mL} / \text{hour}$

5 $\dfrac{80\,\text{mL} \times 60\,\text{minutes}}{50\,\text{minutes}}$

$= 96\,\text{mL} / \text{hour}$

6 $\dfrac{60\,\text{mL} \times 60\,\text{minutes}}{45\,\text{minutes}}$

$= 80\,\text{mL} / \text{hour}$

Activity 10.3

(a) The cyclizine is available as 50 mg/1 mL, and the dose is 50 mg, so the volume to administer would be 1 mL. Therefore, 8 mL – 1 mL = 7 mL water for injection if the cyclizine were to be administered alone.

(b) 10 mg × 3 = 3 mL for the diamorphine. Diamorphine 3 mL + cyclizine 1 mL = 4 mL in total for the drugs; 8 mL – 4 mL for the drugs = 4 mL of water for injection.

(c) 8 mL syringe = 48 mm;

$\dfrac{48\,\text{mm}}{24\,\text{hours}} = 2\,\text{mm} / \text{hour}$

Activity 11.1

1 $\dfrac{50\,\text{mg}}{120\,\text{mg}} \times 5\,\text{mL} = 2.08\,\text{mL}$

2 $\dfrac{35\,\text{mg}}{15\,\text{mg}} \times 5\,\text{mL} = 11.66\,\text{mL}$

3 Weight × dose = 12 kg × 30 mg = 360 mg per daily dose/4 = 90 mg per single dose

4 Weight × dose = 36 kg × 80 mg = 2880 mg per daily dose/4 = 720 mg per single dose

5 2 stone 8 lb = (2 × 14) + 8 = 36 pounds; 36 lb/2.2 kg = 16.36 kg

6 1 kg = 2.2 lb; 6.10 kg = 2.2 × 6.10 = 13.42 lb; 1 lb = 16 oz = 0.42 lb × 16 oz = 6.72 oz. The baby weighs approximately 13 lb 7 oz.

7 Step 1: volume of all drugs per hour = 2 mL per hour + 8 mL every 8 hours + 2 mL every 6 hours: 8 mL/8 hours = 1 mL per hour; 2 mL/6 hours = 0.33 mL every hour = 2 mL + 1 mL + 0.33 mL = 3.33 mL of the drug every hour.

Step 2: $\dfrac{75}{100} \times 45\,\text{mL} = 33.75\,\text{mL} =$ hourly fluid allowance

Step 3: hourly fluid allowance minus the current drug volume = 33.75 mL – 3.33 mL = 30.42 mL. Therefore, the total amount of feed that the child can receive is 30.42 mL every hour.

8 Did you remember to convert the micrograms into milligrams, or milligrams into micrograms so that both units are the same? Change 125 micrograms into milligrams: 125/1000 = 0.125 mg

$\dfrac{0.125\,\text{mg}}{0.5\,\text{mg}} \times 2\,\text{mL} = 0.5\,\text{mL}$

9 $\dfrac{20\,\text{mg}}{50\,\text{mg}} \times 1\,\text{mL} = 0.4\,\text{mL}$

10 BSA = approximately 0.72

11 BSA = approximately 0.69

$$12 \quad \frac{\text{Height} \times \text{weight}}{3600}$$

$$= \frac{87\,\text{cm} \times 14.0\,\text{kg}}{3600} = 03383333$$

Square root = 0.58 m²

Activity 12.1

1 6×150 mL = 900 mL; 900 + 188 + 150 + 1500 mL = 2738 mL Fluid balance = 2738 − 750 mL = 1988 mL

Activity 12.2

1 Fluid balance: 1575 − 1110 = 465 mL
2 Fluid balance: 1125 − 635 = 490 mL
3 Fluid balance: 950 − 900 = 50 mL
4 Fluid balance: 1750 − 500 = 1250 mL
5 Fluid balance: 1150 − 100 = 1050 mL (but where is the urine amount?)
6 Fluid balance: 500 − 900 = −400 mL (a negative amount)

Activity 12.3

1 137 mLs − 18g = 119 mLs
2 Input = 488 mLs
   Output = 360 mLs
   Fluid Balance = 488 − 415 = 73 mLs

Activity 13.1

Step 1 Obese, BMI = 31 kg/m², score = 0
Step 2 Score = 0
Step 3 Score = 2
Step 4 Total = 2, high risk

Step 5 Refer to dietician/nutritional support; set goals; monitor and review.

Activity 14.1

RR: 30 bpm = 3
Sats: 95% = 1
Scale 1
Oxygen therapy = 2
BP: 165 = 0
Pulse: 90 bpm = 0
Alert = 0
Temp: 37.9 Degrees Celsius = 0
Total: 6 and Respiratory Rate scored 3 = inform nurse-in-charge and doctor.

Activity 14.2

RR: 18 bpm = 0
Sats: 98% on Air = 0
BP: 115 = 0
HR: 82 bpm = 0
Alert = 0
Temp: 36.9 degrees Celsius = 0
Total = 0

Activity 14.3

RR: 24 bpm = 2
O_2 Sats: 96% = 0
Scale 1
Oxygen Therapy: Air = 0
BP: 105/50 = 1
Pulse: 120 = 2
ACVPU: Alert = 0
Temp: 38.1 Degrees Celsius = 1
Total: 6 = urgent medical review

Activity 14.4

RR: 25 bpm = 3
O_2 Sats = 94% = 1
Scale 1

Oxygen Therapy: 35% via Venturi Mask = 2
BP: 114/70 = 0
Pulse: 112 bpm = 2
ACVPU: Alert = 0
Temp: 36 degrees Celsius = 1
Total: 9 = emergency medical
assessment

Activity 15.1

Waterlow scores: build, 3; skin type, 1;
sex/age, 2 + 3; malnutrition, A = yes, B
= 2; continence, 1; mobility, 3; special
risks, tissue malnutrition, anaemia = 2;
total Waterlow score, 17 (high risk).

Activity 15.2

Build/Weight for Height: David is obese
(above average BMI) **2**
Skin Type Visual Risk Areas: David has
oedematous skin **1**
Sex/Age: David is an 82-year-old male **1 + 5**
Nutrition: David has not lost weight
recently but has a lack of appetite
presently **1**
Continence: David has no continence
issues **0**
Mobility: David has restricted mobility **3**
Tissue Malnutrition: David is a heavy
smoker **1**
Neurological Deficit: None reported or
observed **0**
Major Surgery or Trauma: None **0**
Medication: David states that he takes
"large white tablets" which he thinks are
some type of steroid. Awaiting his GP
surgery to provide this information. Will add
1 to the score in anticipation, to be reviewed
once this information has been obtained. **1**
What is David's Waterlow score?
15 = High Risk

Activity 16.1

1 2 tablets
2 4 tablets
3 1.5 mL. You need to be aware of
   speed shock.
4 ½ tablet
5 The dose is 1 mL, but you need to
   know when the patient last had this
   injection, as it is to be given once
   every 3 months.
6 3.5 mL. You need to be aware of
   speed shock.

Activity 16.2

1 ½ tablet
2 2½ tablets
3 ½ tablet
4 2 tablets
5 1½ tablets
6 1 tablet

Activity 16.3

All the medications and dosages look
correct for his medical condition (high
blood pressure), but he stated that he
has been taking the medication sublin-
gually (SL) rather than swallowing the
medication (PO), as prescribed.
Therefore, this is the wrong route of
administration.

Activity 17.1

1 Budget for education: £2200 per
   annum
   Registered general nurses:
   venepuncture, 6 × £57.50 = £345;
   male catheterisation, 6 × £57.50 =
   £345

Care assistants: catheter care, 24 × £57.50 = £1380; Basic Clinical Skills 1 × £400 (12 staff) = £400 £345 + £345 + £1380 + £400 = Total: £2470; this exceeds the education budget by £270. (2470 − 2200 = 270)

2 6 registered general nurses:24 care assistants:12 customer services staff = 6:24:12 = 1:4:2

Activity 17.2

1 B and C 20/100 = 0.2
   0.2 × £600 000 = 120 000
2 42 000
   5/100 = 0.05
   0.05 × 480 000 = 24 000
   480 000 + 24 000 = 504 000
   504 000/12 = 42 000.

Activity 17.3

1 £145 billion
2 Social Protection, £240 billion
3 £34 billion
4 £145 billion − £34 billion = £111 billion

Activity 17.4

1 What is the percentage difference for expenditure on Social Protection from 2016/2017 to 2019/2020? 275.3 − 240 = 35.3
   (a) $\dfrac{35.3}{240} \times 100 = 14.7$ = Increased by 15%
2 What is the percentage difference for expenditure on Health from 2016/2017 to 2019/2020? 164.1 − 145 = 19.1

(b) $\dfrac{19.1}{145} \times 100 = 13.1$ = Increased by 13%

3 What is the total percentage difference for expenditure on education from 2016/2017 to 1019/2020? 92.4 − 102 = −9.6
   c $\dfrac{-9.6}{102} \times 100 = -9.4$ = Decreased by 9.4%

4 What is the total percentage difference for expenditure on defence from 2016/2017 to 2019/2010? 42.2 − 46 = −3.8
   $\dfrac{-3.8}{46} \times 100 = -8.2 = -8\%$

Activity 18.1

1 Near Misses
2 TRALI = Transfusion-related acute lung injury = 3 × 3397 = 10 191 (n number = 3397)

Activity 18.2

Sodium: 145 mmol/L (133–146 mmol/L) = acceptable range
Bicarbonate: 30 mmol/L (22–26 mmol/L) = outside of acceptable range

Activity 18.3

1 Metabolic alkalosis
2 Respiratory acidosis

Activity 18.4

1 Swindon – 528
2 Swindon – 552
3 Cheltenham – 251

4 Stroud – 225

5 Reduced figures on 8 January 2021 from the 1 January 2021:
- Gloucester (496 down to 491)
- Sedgemoor 481 down to 424)
- Somerset West and Taunton (449 down to 380)
- Cotswold (288 down to 258)
- Stroud (258 down to 225)

6 1 January 2021 mean average: 596/17 = 350.6 = 351
8 January 2021 mean average: 6502/17 = 382.4 = 382

Activity 18.5

1 a) 400 000 000 × £2.23 = £892 000 000

b) 100 000 000 × £2.23 = £223 000 000

2 a) 56 000 000 × £28.00 = £1 568 000 000

b) Nothing, as Australia did not order any Moderna vaccine initially.

3 a) £14.80 × 20 000 000 = 1 776 000 000 × 2 as two doses asked for = £3 552 000 000

b) £14.80 × 40 000 = 592 000 000 × 2 as two doses asked for = £1 184 000 000

4 Vaccine = 0.5 mLs. 10 doses per vial = 10 × 0.5 = 5 mLs

Activity 19.1

1 $\frac{50\,mg}{80\,mg} \times 2\,mL = 1.25\,mL$

2 $\frac{300\,mg}{500\,mg} \times 100\,mL = 60\,mL$

3 $\frac{60\,mg}{30\,mg} = 2\,tablets$

4 Weight × dose = 2.5 kg × 10 mg = 25 mg daily. Divide this by 3 to get the 8-hourly dose = 8.3 mg

5 $\frac{1000\,mL}{12\,hours} \times \frac{20\,drops\,/\,mL}{60\,minutes} = 27.77$
= 28 drops per minute (to nearest whole drop)

6 (a) $\frac{30\,000\,units}{25\,000\,units} \times 5\,mL = 6\,mL$

(b) Dilutant (48 mL) minus the volume of drug (6 mL) = 42.0 mL; this makes sure that we have a total of 48 mL in the syringe and not 48 plus 6 mL. This would make 54 mL, which is too much and a drug error.

7 $\frac{450\,mL}{4\,hours} \times \frac{15\,drops\,/\,mL}{60\,minutes} = 28.125$
= 28 drops per minute

8 $\frac{600\ mL}{20\ drops\ per\ minute} \times \frac{15\ drops/mL}{60\ minutes} = 7.5$ (7½ hours)

9 $\frac{75\,mg}{100\,mg} \times 2\,mL = 1.5\,mL$

10 $\frac{225\,mg}{150\,mg} = 1.5 = 1½\,tablets$

Activity 19.2

1 $\frac{50\ mg}{25\ mg} \times 10\ mL = 20\ mL$

2 $\frac{40\ mg}{50\ mg} \times 5\ mL = 4\ mL$

3 $\frac{20000}{4000} \times 5\ mL = 25\ mL$

4 $\frac{80\ mg}{50\ mg} \times 2\ mL = 3.2\ mL$

5 $\frac{2000\ microgram}{300\ microgram} \times 3\ mL = 19.99\ mL$

6 6.66 mLs

7 0.83 mLs

8 1.75 mLs
9 0.75 mLs
10 1.6 mLs

Activity 19.3

1 500 mcg = 0.5 mg/0.5 mLs.
Therefore, 0.5 mLs.

2 $\dfrac{\text{VoL}}{\text{TIME}} \times \dfrac{\text{Drops per mL}}{\text{Mins per hour}} \dfrac{1000}{5} \times \dfrac{20}{60}$
= 66.666 = 67 dpm

3 $\dfrac{\text{WHAT YOU WANT}}{\text{WHAT YOU'VE GOT}} \dfrac{500}{500} = 1$ tablet

4 Weight (kg) × Dose
120 × 20 = 2400 mg (Daily dose)
Single Dose (4 hourly) =
$\dfrac{2400}{6} = 400$ mLs

5 4.5 mls/hr for 3 hours = 13.5 mLs
4.0 mls/hr for 2 hours = 8.0 mLs
2.0 mls/hr for 2 hours = 4.0 mLs
3.0 mls/hr for 1 hour = 3.0 mLs
3.5 mls/hr for 4 hours = 14.0 mLs
= 42.5 Units

6 2 mg = 1 mL
2 mg = 1 mL
1 mg = 0.50 mLs
0.5 mg = 0.25 mL = 2.75 mL

7 $\dfrac{\text{Vol}}{\text{Time}} \times \dfrac{\text{Drops per mL}}{\text{Mins per hour}} \dfrac{1000}{10} \times \dfrac{20}{60} =$
33.33 = 33 drops/m

8 If a type J cylinder runs at 8 litres per minute, how many hours supply are there left? **NOTE**: Formula = cylinder capacity (litres) divided by flow rate (litres per minute) divided by 60 = hours supply.
6800 divided by 8.0 divided by 60 = 14.2 hours supply in the cylinder.

Activity 19.4

1 a) How many mLs of Alfentanil do you draw up?
$\dfrac{\text{WHAT YOU WANT}}{\text{WHAT YOU'VE GOT}} \times \text{VOL} = \dfrac{2\text{ mg}}{5\text{ mg}} \times 1 =$
0.4 mLs

b) How many mLs of saline do you require to make the solution up to 50 mLs?
50 mls – 0.4 mls = 49.6 mLs OF DILUTANT

c) How many mLs/hr do you need to set the pump?
$\dfrac{\text{WHAT YOU WANT}}{\text{WHAT YOU'VE GOT}} \times \text{VOL} = \dfrac{0.2\text{ mg}}{2\text{ mg}} \times 50 =$
5 mLs/hr

2 $\dfrac{\text{WHAT YOU WANT}}{\text{WHAT YOU'VE GOT}} \times \text{VOL} =$
$\dfrac{40\text{ micrograms}}{50\text{ micrograms}} \times 2$ mls = 1.6 mLs

3 Weight × Dose = 2.2 kg × 0. 4 mg = 0.88 mg
Intramuscular

4 a) What dose is prescribed?
Weight (kg) × Dose
1.2 kg × 50 mg = 210 mg

b) It comes as 600 mg in 4 mls of water. How much do you give?
$\dfrac{\text{WHAT YOU WANT}}{\text{WHAT YOU'VE GOT}} \times \text{VOL} \dfrac{210\text{ mg}}{600\text{ mg}} \times$
4 mLs = 1.4 mls

5 a) What is the prescribed dose?
Change grams into kg = 975/1000 = 0.975
Weight (kg) × Dose
0.975 × 15 mg = 14.625 mg

b) How much is going to be infused?

$$\frac{\text{WHAT YOU WANT}}{\text{WHAT YOU'VE GOT}} \times \text{VOL} \frac{14.625 \text{ mg}}{50 \text{ mg}} \times$$

10 mLs = 2925 mLs

6 a) What amount is prescribed?

Change grams into kg = 650/1000
= 0.65 kg

Weight (kg) × Dose

1.65 g × 50 mg = 32.5 mg

b) Cefotaxime comes as 500 mg in 5 mls of water. What amount do you give?

$$\frac{\text{WHAT YOU WANT}}{\text{WHAT YOU'VE GOT}} \times \text{VOL} \frac{32.5 \text{ mg}}{500 \text{ mg}} \times$$

5 mLs = 0.325 mLs

7 a) How much is prescribed?

Weight (kg) × Dose

3.64 g × 7.5 mg = 27.3 mg

b) It comes as 50 mg in 10 mls, how much is given?

$$\frac{\text{WHAT YOU WANT}}{\text{WHAT YOU'VE GOT}} \times \text{VOL} \frac{27.3 \text{ mg}}{50 \text{ mg}}$$

× 10 mls = 5.46 mLs

8 a) How much is prescribed?

Weight (kg) × Dose 4.5 kg × 50 mg
= 225 mg

b) $\frac{\text{WHAT YOU WANT}}{\text{WHAT YOU'VE GOT}} \times \text{VOL} \frac{225 \text{ mg}}{250 \text{ mg}}$

× 5 mLs = 4.5 mLs

9 a) Weight (kg) × Dose

3.1 kg × 2 mg = 6.2 mg

Use this formula:

amount in mgs (your answer from 9a) × by 1000 (to convert to mcg/kg/hour) divide by 50 (mLs of fluid in the syringe), then divide by infants weight × by rate infusion is prescribed at.

Mg × 1000 ÷ 50 ÷ weight × rate = mcg per kg per hour

b) The pump is running at 0.5 ml/hr. How many mcg/kg/hr is the baby receiving?

6.2 mg × 1000/50/3.1 kg × 0.5 mls
= 20 mcg/kg/hr

10 a) Work out dose for the same baby (3.1 kg).

Weight (kg) × Dose = 3.1 kg × 120 mg = 372 mg

Use this formula;

amount in mgs (your answer from 10a) × by 1000 (to convert to mcg/kg/hour) divide by 50 (mLs of fluid in the syringe), then divide by infant's weight, then divide by 60 to convert to per minute × by rate infusion is prescribed at = mcg/kg/minute.

Mg × 1000 ÷ 50 ÷ weight ÷ 60 × rate = mcg per kg per minute

b) The pump is running at 0.25 mL/hr. How many mcg/kg/minute is the baby receiving?

372 mg × 1000/50/3.1 kg/60 × 0.25 mLs/hr = 10 mcg/kg/min

Activity 19.5

1 $\frac{\text{WYW}}{\text{WYG}} \times \text{Vol} \frac{6.5 \text{ mg}}{2.5 \text{ mg}} \times 1 \text{ mL} =$
2.6 mL

2 $\frac{\text{WYW}}{\text{WYG}} \times \text{Vol} \frac{7.5 \text{ mg}}{5 \text{ mg}} \times 2 \text{ mL} = 3 \text{ mL}$

3 1 week = 7 days

56 mg = 7 days dosage

56/7 = 8 mg

Therefore, patient requires 8 mg per day.

NOTE: I can reverse check that my answer is right: 8 mg × 7 days = 56 mg

4 $\dfrac{WYW}{WYG} \times Vol \dfrac{15\ mg}{50\ mg} \times 5\ mL = 1.5\ mLs$

Activity 19.6

1 $\dfrac{WYW}{WYW} \times Vol \dfrac{40\ mg}{5\ mg} \times 1\ mL = 8\ mLs$

2 500 mcg + 500 mcg = 2 ampoules each dose

3 2500/24 =104.166 = 104 mLs/hour

INPUT	INPUT	OUTPUT
80 mL Tea	500 mL IV N/ Saline	150 mL Urine
100 mL Milk		200 mL Urine
50 mL Juice		70 mL Urine
200 mL Soup		250 mL Urine
70 mL Tea		
180 mL cocoa		500 mL Urine

4 ANSWER: INPUT: 680 mL + 500 mL = 1180 mL
OUTPUT: 1170 mLs
Input 1180 minus output 1170 = 10 mL = positive output, i.e., input is slightly more than output.

Activity 19.7

1 7.5 mg = 3 tablets × 7 days (1 week) = 21
10 mg = 4 tablets × 14 days (2 weeks) = 56
21 + 56 = 77 tablets (enough tablets for 3 weeks' supply)

2 Change grams into mg = 1 g = 1000 mg
$\dfrac{1000}{275} \times 3\ mls = 10.9\ mls$

3 11.5 kg × 100 = 1150
Divide this by 2 (two divided doses) = 575 mg

4 Change 0.025 mg into micrograms = 0.025 × 1000 = 25
$\dfrac{25}{50} = 0.5 \times 14$ days) = 7 tablets

5 Change micrograms into mg = 100 micrograms/1000 = 0.1 mg
0.1 × 28 = 2.8 mg

Activity 20.1

24.4 kg/m^2 makes this person normal weight.

Activity 20.2

1 $\dfrac{93.5}{1.75 \times 1.75} = 3.0625 = 30.5$ kg/m^2 Obese

2 $\dfrac{79}{1.67 \times 1.67} = 2.7889 = 28.3$ kg/m^2 Overweight

3 $\dfrac{47.2}{1.84 \times 1.84} = 3.3856 = 13.9$ kg/m^2 Underweight

4 $\dfrac{72.6}{1.57 \times 1.57} = 2.4649 = 29.4$ kg/m^2 Overweight

5 $\dfrac{80}{1.54 \times 1.54} = 2.3716 = 33.7$ kg/m^2 Obese

6 $\dfrac{62}{1.82 \times 1.82} = 3.3124 = 18.7$ kg/m^2 Normal

7 $\dfrac{88}{1.61 \times 1.61} = 2.5921 = 33.9$ kg/m^2 Obese

8 $\dfrac{78}{1.86 \times 1.86} = 3.4596 = 22.5$ kg/m^2 Normal

9 $\dfrac{65}{1.66 \times 1.66} = 2.7556 = 23.5 \text{ kg/m}^2$

Normal

10 $\dfrac{79}{1.86 \times 1.86} = 3.4596 = 22.8 \text{ kg/m}^2$

Normal

Activity 20.3

Patient A weighs 105 kg and has a height of 1.65 m. First, square the height: 1.65 × 1.65 = 2.7225. Next, divide the weight by the squared height and round up your answer:

105 / 2.7225 = 38.56

= 38.6 kg / m^2

Therefore, the patient falls into the obese category (BMI 30–39.9 kg/m^2).

Activity 20.4

Sorry – I don't know your weight and height to give an answer to this question! How many of you turned to this answer section to check your answer?!

Activity 20.5

$\dfrac{79 \text{ kg} - 75 \text{ kg}}{79 \text{kg}} \times 100 = 5$

Or/

1 79 kg – 75 kg = 4 kg

2 4/79 = 0.05

3 × 100 = 5 (to get the percentage amount)

Therefore, Ernest has lost 5% of his body weight

Activity 21.1

QUESTION	WORKING OUT	ANSWER
1 Convert 7.8 kg to grams	Larger unit kg to smaller unit g = × 1000 7.8 × 1000 =	7800 grams
2 Convert 7555 mcg to mg	Smaller unit mcg to larger unit mg = /1000 7555/1000 =	7.555 mg
3 Convert 1.7 litres to mL	Larger unit l to smaller unit mL = × 1000 1.7 × 1000 =	1700 mL
4 Convert 43 mL to litres	Smaller unit mL to larger unit l = /1000 43/1000 =	0.043 litres
5 Convert 3.56 g to mg	Larger unit g to smaller unit mg = × 1000 3.56 × 1000 =	3560 mg
6 Convert 25 mcg to mg	Smaller unit mcg to larger unit mg = /1000 25 / 1000 =	0.025 mg

QUESTION	WORKING OUT	ANSWER
7 Convert 777 mg to grams	Smaller unit mg to larger unit g = /1000 777/1000 =	0.777 g
8 Convert 0.5 litres to mL	Larger unit l to smaller unit mL = × 1000 0.5 × 1000 =	500 mL
9 Convert 451 mL to litres	Smaller unit mL to larger unit l = /1000 451/1000 =	0.451 litre
10 Convert 1.9 metres to centimetres	Larger unit m to smaller unit cm = 1.9 × 1000 =	1900 cm
11 A patient has been prescribed 300 mg of a drug every 4 hours. The stock tablets on hand are 150 mg. How many tablets do you need to give to the patient in a day?	24 hours 4 hourly = Means that the drug needs to be administered 6 times per day. 300 mg (prescribed dose) × 6 = 1800 mg per day. $$\frac{WYW}{WYG} = \frac{1800 \text{ mg}}{150 \text{ mg}} =$$ Don't forget to divide your answer by 6 as tablets to be administered every 4 hours.	12 tablets per day /6 = 2 tablets
12 A drug error has been made. 0.1 mL of a drug has been administered to a patient when it should have been 0.01 mL. How many times too much is this?	This is a factor of 10, meaning the decimal point in 0.1 should have been moved once to the left. Or, 0.1/10 = 0.01 mL =	10 times too much
13 A patient requires 500 mcg of a drug. You have an ampoule of the drug presented as 1 mg in 1 mL. How many mLs do you give?	First convert the 500 mcg into mg = 500/1000 = 0.5 mg. Then use formula= $$\frac{WYW}{WYG} \times VOL \; \frac{0.5 \text{ mg}}{1.0 \text{ mg}} \times 1 \text{ mL} =$$	0.5 mLs

QUESTION	WORKING OUT	ANSWER
14 35 units of insulin has been prescribed. It is dispensed as 100 units in 1 mL. How many mLs do you administer?	$\dfrac{WYW}{WYG} \times VOL$ $\dfrac{35 \text{ units}}{100 \text{ units}} \times 1 =$	0.35 mLs
15 A patient is given 2 litres of 0.45% saline. How many grams of sodium will the patient receive?	Change 2 litres into mL = 2l = 2000 mLs $\dfrac{2000 \times 0.45}{100} =$	9 g
16 A patient weighs 60 kg and requires 40 mcg/kg of a drug. **a** How many mcg are required? **b** How many mg is this?	Weight × Dose = 60 kg × 40 mcg = Change mcg into mg = 2400/1000 =	2400 mcg 2.4 mg
17 How many grams of medication do you have in 15g of 12% w/w ointment?	$15 \times \dfrac{12}{100} =$	1.8 g
18 A patient has been prescribed ibuprofen 5 mg/mg/dose. She weighs 65 kg. Calculate how much ibuprofen you need to administer.	Weight × dose 65 kg × 5 mg =	325 mg
19 A patient has been prescribed 20 mL of lactulose b.d. How many full days supply of lactulose is there in a 500 mL bottle?	First remember b.d = twice a day, therefore patient requires 40 mLs of lactulose per day. How many lots of 40 mLs can I get out of a 500 mL bottle?	The bottle of lactulose will last 12 days as there are 12 lots of 40 mL in the 500 mL bottle (with 20 mLs left over).

QUESTION	WORKING OUT	ANSWER
20 A patient is prescribed 9 mg of Morphine. Stock solution is 15 mg in 1 mL. How much do you administer?	$\dfrac{WYW}{WYG \times VOL}$ $\dfrac{9\ mg}{15\ mg} \times 1 = mL$	0.6 mL

Chapter 21

Knowledge test 1

1 Waterlow, Walter Jones: score = 13
2 Jane Fielding
  RR: 18 bpm = 0
  Scale 1
  SpO2: 99% Air = 0
  BP: 130/80 = 0
  HR: 80 bpm = 0
  Neuro: Alert = 0
  Temp: 37.1 degrees Celsius
  Total: 0
3 $\dfrac{35\,mg}{60\,mg} \times 1\,mL = 0.58\,mL$
4 $\dfrac{27\,mg}{30\,mg} \times 10\,mL = 9\,mL$
5 **(a)** Weight × dose = 100 kg × 10 mg = 1000 mg

  (b) Change 4 g into milligrams
  = 4000 mg
  $\dfrac{1000\,mg}{4000\,mg} \times 400\,mL$
  = 100 mL / hour

6 **(a)** $\dfrac{15\,mg}{20\,mg} \times 2\,mL = 1.5\,mL$

  (b) $\dfrac{15\,mg}{3\,mg\,/\,min} = 5\,minutes$

7 $\dfrac{6\,mg}{15\,mg} \times 1\,mL = 0.4\,mL$

8 First change 1.5 g into milligrams
  $= 1500\,mg\ \dfrac{1500\,mg}{500\,mg} \times 10\,mL$
  $= 30\,mL$
9 **(a)** Weight × dose = 1.2 kg × 2.5 mg = 3 mg
  (b) $\dfrac{3\,mg}{5\,mg} \times 5\,mL =$
  3 mL over 10 minutes
10 **(a)** Weight × dose = 3.4 kg × 50 mg = 170 mg
  (b) $\dfrac{170\,mg}{600\,mg} \times 4\,mL = 1.13\,mL$

Knowledge test 2

1 MUST, Max Norman: 33 kg/m^2 = obese. Score on the MUST BMI chart = 0.
2 Robert Hayes
  RR: 36 bpm = 3
  Scale 1
  SpO2: 89% Air = 3
  BP: 108/70 = 1
  HR: 129 bpm = 2
  Neuro: Alert = 0
  Temp: 38.4 Degrees Celsius = 1
  Total: 10 Patient requires an emergency medical assessment and continuous monitoring
3 $\dfrac{75\,mg}{50\,mg} \times 1\,mL = 1.5\,mL$
4 First change 75 micrograms into milligrams = 0.075 mg

$$\frac{0.075\,mg}{0.1\,mg} \times 1\,mL = 0.75\,mL$$

5 $\dfrac{275\,micrograms}{500\,micrograms} \times 2\,mL = 1.1\,mL$

6 First change 1 mg into micrograms
= 1000 micrograms

$$\frac{500\,micrograms}{1000\,micrograms} \times 1\,mL = 0.5\,mL$$

7 Weight × dose = 90 kg × 80 mg =
7200 mg (daily dose)
Single dose (given 6 hourly):

$$\frac{7200\,mg}{4} = 1800\,mg, \text{ or } 1.8\,grams$$

8 (a) Weight × dose = 4.2 kg ×
50 mg/kg = 210 mg

(b) $\dfrac{210\,mg}{600\,mg} \times 4\,mL = 1.4\,mL$

9 Step 1: establish how much fluid
left to infuse = 2000 mL − 700 mL
= 1300 mL
Step 2: establish how much time is
left to infuse = 24 hours − 10 hours
= 14 hours
Step 3:

$$\frac{1300\,mL}{14\,hours} \times \frac{20\,drops\,/\,mL}{60\,minutes}$$

= 30.9 = 31 drops per minute

10 3 mL × 1 hour = 3.0 mL
3.5 mL × 2 hours = 7.0 mL
2 mL × 2 hours = 4.0 mL
2.5 mL × 2 hours = 5.0 mL
4 mL × 1 hour = 4.0 mL
23.0 units of Actrapid have been
received in total.

Knowledge test 3

1 Waterlow, Violet Simms: score = 20,
high risk

2 Simon Patrick
RR: 20 bpm = 0
Scale 1
Sp02: 96% on Air = 0
BP: 120/71 = 0
HR: 100 bpm = 1
Neuro: Alert = 0
Temp: 38.0 Degrees Celsius = 0
Total = 1

3 $\dfrac{22\,mg}{20\,mg} \times 2\,mL = 2.2\,mL$

4 $\dfrac{30\,mg}{20\,mg} \times 2\,mL = 3\,mL$

5 $\dfrac{20\,mg}{10\,mg} \times 10\,mL = 20\,mL$

6 (a) $\dfrac{2.5\,mg}{5\,mg} \times 10\,mL = 5\,mL$

(b) $\dfrac{2.5\,mg}{1\,mg\,/\,min} = 2.5\,minutes$

7 3 mg is given in 1 mL, 6 mg in
2 mL and 12 mg in 4 mL
1 mL + 2 mL + 4 mL = total volume
of 7 mL

8 (a) Weight × dose = 3.1 kg × 2 mg
= 6.2 mg
Use this formula:
Dose (mg) × 1000 ÷ 50 ÷
weight (kg) × rate (mL / hour)
= micrograms / kg per hour

(b) 6.2 × 1000 ÷ 50 ÷ 3.1 × 0.5 =
20 micrograms/kg per hour

9 $\dfrac{500\,mL}{35\,drops\,/\,minute} \times \dfrac{15\,drops\,/\,mL}{60\,minutes}$

= 3.57 = just over 3‰ hours

10 (i) 6 micrograms = 0.006 mg ×
60 minutes = 0.36 mg/hour

(ii) Weight × dose = 75 kg ×
0.36 mg = 27 mg

(iii) $\dfrac{27\,mg}{150\,mg} \times 500\,mL$

= 90 mL / hour

Knowledge test 4

1 MUST, Sarah Hann: 17 kg/m^2.
   Score on the MUST BMI chart = 2.

2 Lesley David
   RR: 10 bpm = 1
   Scale 2
   SpO2: 90% on Air = 0
   BP: 99/60 = 2
   HR: 51 bpm = 0
   Neuro: Confused = 3
   Temp: 37 Degrees Celsius = 0
   Total: 6 Inform nurse-in-charge
   and Doctor as patient is scoring 3 in
   Neuro obs = newly confused

3 $\dfrac{200\,mg}{600\,mg} \times 10\,mL = 3.33\,mL$

4 First change 1 g into milligrams =
   1000 mg

   a $\dfrac{500\,mg}{1000\,mg} \times 20\,mL = 10\,mL$

   b $\dfrac{500\,mg}{4\,mg\,/\,min} = 125\,minutes$

   c **Step 1:** add up total volume of
      fluids = 10 mL vancomycin +
      500 mL sodium chloride =
      510 mL
      Step 2: change the rate per
      minute into an hourly rate =

4 mg/minute × 60 minutes =
240 mg/hour

Step 3: $\dfrac{\dfrac{240\,mg\,/\,hour}{500\,mg}}{} \times 510\,mL$

$= 244.8\,mL\,/\,hour$

5 $\dfrac{350\,mL}{3\,hours} \times \dfrac{15\,drops\,/\,mL}{60\,minutes} = 29.16$

$= 29\,drops\,per\,minute$

6 $\dfrac{5\,mg}{10\,mg} \times 10\,mL = 5\,mL$

7 $\dfrac{1000\,mL}{20\,drops\,/\,minute} \times \dfrac{15\,drops\,/\,mL}{60\,minutes}$
   $= 12.5 = 12\%\,hours$

8 (a) First change grams into
      kilograms = 0.975 kg Weight ×
      dose = 0.975 kg × 15 mg =
      14.625 mg

   (b) $\dfrac{14.625\,mg}{50\,mg} \times 10\,mL$

      $= 2.925\,mL$

9 (a) First change 500 micrograms
      into milligrams = 0.5 mg Weight
      × dose = 65 kg × 0.5 mg =
      32.5 mg/hour

   (b) $\dfrac{32.5\,mg\,/\,hour}{250\,mg} \times 100\,mL$

      $= 13\,mL\,/\,hour$

10 Weight × dose = 70 kg × 1.5 mg =
    1 05 mg

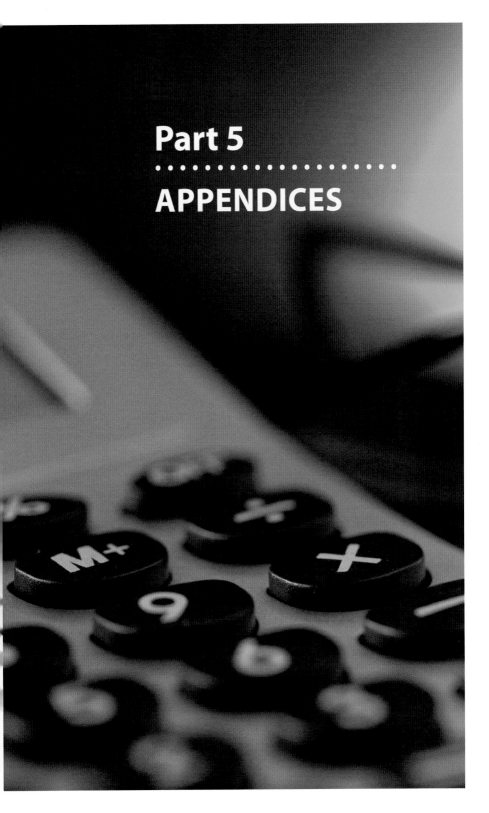

Part 5
. . . .
APPENDICES

Appendix 1

FLUID CHART

Calculation Skills for Nurses, Second Edition. Claire Boyd.
© 2022 John Wiley & Sons Ltd. Published 2022 by John Wiley & Sons Ltd.

FLUID CHART

24h Fluid Record	NO:
	Surname:
Date: _____ . _____ . _____	Forenames:
Previous Day's Balance: _____ mL	Dob:
	Ward:

Time   Input Route (mL)   Output Route (mL)

Hour Ending	Oral	Enteral Tube			TOTAL	Urine	Gastric/ Vomit			TOTAL
08.00										
09.00										
10.00										
11.00										
12.00										
13.00										
14.00										
15.00										
16.00										
17.00										
18.00										
19.00										
20.00										
21.00										
22.00										
23.00										
24.00										
01.00										
02.00										
03.00										
04.00										
05.00										
06.00										
07.00										
24h Total										
					24h Input					**24h Output**

24h Balance =   mL

Source: reproduced here with permission from North Bristol NHS Trust and University Hospitals Bristol NHS Foundation Trust.

Appendix 2

. . . .

MALNUTRITION UNIVERSAL SCREENING TOOL

Calculation Skills for Nurses, Second Edition. Claire Boyd.
© 2022 John Wiley & Sons Ltd. Published 2022 by John Wiley & Sons Ltd.

'Malnutrition Universal Screening Tool'

BAPEN is registered charity number 1023927 www.bapen.org.uk

'MUST'

'MUST' is a five-step screening tool to identify **adults,** who are malnourished, at risk of malnutrition (undernutrition), or obese. It also includes management guidelines which can be used to develop a care plan.

It is for use in hospitals, community and other care settings and can be used by all care workers.

This guide contains:

- A flow chart showing the 5 steps to use for screening and management
- BMI chart
- Weight loss tables
- Alternative measurements when BMI cannot be obtained by measuring weight and height.

The 5 'MUST' Steps

Step 1
Measure height and weight to get a BMI score using chart provided. *If unable to obtain height and weight, use the alternative procedures shown in this guide.*

Step 2
Note percentage unplanned weight loss and score using tables provided.

Step 3
Establish acute disease effect and score.

Step 4
Add scores from steps 1, 2 and 3 together to obtain overall risk of malnutrition.

Step 5
Use management guidelines and/or local policy to develop care plan.

Please refer to *The 'MUST' Explanatory Booklet* for more information when weight and height cannot be measured, and when screening patient groups in which extra care in interpretation is needed (e.g. those with fluid disturbances, plaster casts, amputations, critical illness and pregnant or lactating women). The booklet can also be used for training. See *The 'MUST' Report* for supporting evidence. Please note that 'MUST' has not been designed to detect deficiencies or excessive intakes of vitamins and minerals and is of **use only in adults.**

© BAPEN

Step 1 – BMI score (& BMI)

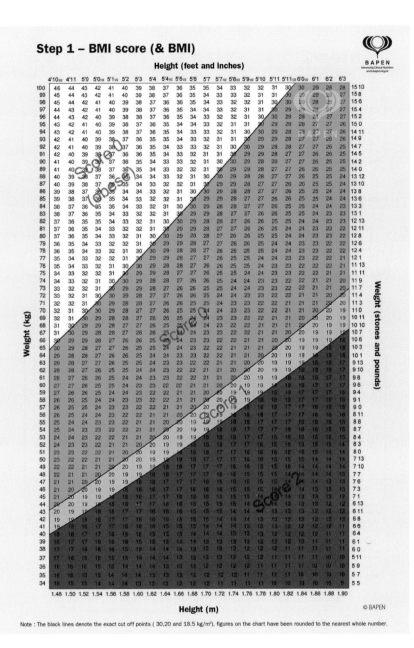

Height (feet and inches)

Weight (kg) / **Weight (stones and pounds)**

Height (m)

© BAPEN

Note : The black lines denote the exact cut off points (30,20 and 18.5 kg/m²), figures on the chart have been rounded to the nearest whole number.

+ 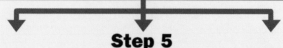 **Step 3**
BAPEN

Step 1
BMI score

BMI kg/m²	Score
>20 (>30 Obese)	= 0
18.5-20	= 1
<18.5	= 2

If unable to obtain height and weight, see reverse for alternative measurements and use of subjective criteria

Step 2
Weight loss score

Unplanned weight loss in past 3-6 months

%	Score
<5	= 0
5-10	= 1
>10	= 2

Step 3
Acute disease effect score

If patient is acutely ill **and** there has been or is likely to be no nutritional intake for >5 days
Score 2

Acute disease effect is unlikely to apply outside hospital. See 'MUST' Explanatory Booklet for further information

Step 4
Overall risk of malnutrition

Add Scores together to calculate overall risk of malnutrition
Score 0 Low Risk   Score 1 Medium Risk   Score 2 or more High Risk

Step 5
Management guidelines

0
Low Risk
Routine clinical care

- Repeat screening
  Hospital – weekly
  Care Homes – monthly
  Community – annually
  for special groups
  e.g. those >75 yrs

1
Medium Risk
Observe

- Document dietary intake for 3 days
- If adequate – little concern and repeat screening
  - Hospital – weekly
  - Care Home – at least monthly
  - Community – at least every 2-3 months
- If inadequate – clinical concern – follow local policy, set goals, improve and increase overall nutritional intake, monitor and review care plan regularly

2 or more
High Risk
Treat*

- Refer to dietitian, Nutritional Support Team or implement local policy
- Set goals, improve and increase overall nutritional intake
- Monitor and review care plan
  Hospital – weekly
  Care Home – monthly
  Community – monthly

* Unless detrimental or no benefit is expected from nutritional support e.g. imminent death.

All risk categories:
- Treat underlying condition and provide help and advice on food choices, eating and drinking when necessary.
- Record malnutrition risk category.
- Record need for special diets and follow local policy.

Obesity:
- Record presence of obesity. For those with underlying conditions, these are generally controlled before the treatment of obesity.

Re-assess subjects identified at risk as they move through care settings
See The 'MUST' Explanatory Booklet for further details and The 'MUST' Report for supporting evidence.

Step 2 – Weight loss score

BAPEN
Advancing Clinical Nutrition
www.bapen.org.uk

Weight before weight loss (kg)

	SCORE 0 Wt Loss <5%	SCORE 1 Wt Loss 5-10%	SCORE 2 Wt Loss >10%
34 kg	<1.70	1.70 – 3.40	>3.40
36 kg	<1.80	1.80 – 3.60	>3.60
38 kg	<1.90	1.90 – 3.80	>3.80
40 kg	<2.00	2.00 – 4.00	>4.00
42 kg	<2.10	2.10 – 4.20	>4.20
44 kg	<2.20	2.20 – 4.40	>4.40
46 kg	<2.30	2.30 – 4.60	>4.60
48 kg	<2.40	2.40 – 4.80	>4.80
50 kg	<2.50	2.50 – 5.00	>5.00
52 kg	<2.60	2.60 – 5.20	>5.20
54 kg	<2.70	2.70 – 5.40	>5.40
56 kg	<2.80	2.80 – 5.60	>5.60
58 kg	<2.90	2.90 – 5.80	>5.80
60 kg	<3.00	3.00 – 6.00	>6.00
62 kg	<3.10	3.10 – 6.20	>6.20
64 kg	<3.20	3.20 – 6.40	>6.40
66 kg	<3.30	3.30 – 6.60	>6.60
68 kg	<3.40	3.40 – 6.80	>6.80
70 kg	<3.50	3.50 – 7.00	>7.00
72 kg	<3.60	3.60 – 7.20	>7.20
74 kg	<3.70	3.70 – 7.40	>7.40
76 kg	<3.80	3.80 – 7.60	>7.60
78 kg	<3.90	3.90 – 7.80	>7.80
80 kg	<4.00	4.00 – 8.00	>8.00
82 kg	<4.10	4.10 – 8.20	>8.20
84 kg	<4.20	4.20 – 8.40	>8.40
86 kg	<4.30	4.30 – 8.60	>8.60
88 kg	<4.40	4.40 – 8.80	>8.80
90 kg	<4.50	4.50 – 9.00	>9.00
92 kg	<4.60	4.60 – 9.20	>9.20
94 kg	<4.70	4.70 – 9.40	>9.40
96 kg	<4.80	4.80 – 9.60	>9.60
98 kg	<4.90	4.90 – 9.80	>9.80
100 kg	<5.00	5.00 – 10.00	>10.00
102 kg	<5.10	5.10 – 10.20	>10.20
104 kg	<5.20	5.20 – 10.40	>10.40
106 kg	<5.30	5.30 – 10.60	>10.60
108 kg	<5.40	5.40 – 10.80	>10.80
110 kg	<5.50	5.50 – 11.00	>11.00
112 kg	<5.60	5.60 – 11.20	>11.20
114 kg	<5.70	5.70 – 11.40	>11.40
116 kg	<5.80	5.80 – 11.60	>11.60
118 kg	<5.90	5.90 – 11.80	>11.80
120 kg	<6.00	6.00 – 12.00	>12.00
122 kg	<6.10	6.10 – 12.20	>12.20
124 kg	<6.20	6.20 – 12.40	>12.40
126 kg	<6.30	6.30 – 12.60	>12.60

Weight before weight loss (st lb)

	SCORE 0 Wt Loss <5%	SCORE 1 Wt Loss 5-10%	SCORE 2 Wt Loss >10%
5st 4lb	<4lb	4lb – 7lb	>7lb
5st 7lb	<4lb	4lb – 8lb	>8lb
5st 11lb	<4lb	4lb – 8lb	>8lb
6st	<4lb	4lb – 8lb	>8lb
6st 4lb	<4lb	4lb – 9lb	>9lb
6st 7lb	<5lb	5lb – 9lb	>9lb
6st 11lb	<5lb	5lb – 10lb	>10lb
7st	<5lb	5lb – 10lb	>10lb
7st 4lb	<5lb	5lb – 10lb	>10lb
7st 7lb	<5lb	5lb – 11lb	>11lb
7st 11lb	<5lb	5lb – 11lb	>11lb
8st	<6lb	6lb – 11lb	>11lb
8st 4lb	<6lb	6lb – 12lb	>12lb
8st 7lb	<6lb	6lb – 12lb	>12lb
8st 11lb	<6lb	6lb – 12lb	>12lb
9st	<6lb	6lb – 13lb	>13lb
9st 4lb	<7lb	7lb – 13lb	>13lb
9st 7lb	<7lb	7lb – 13lb	>13lb
9st 11lb	<7lb	7lb – 1st 0lb	>1st 0lb
10st	<7lb	7lb – 1st 0lb	>1st 0lb
10st 4lb	<7lb	7lb – 1st 0lb	>1st 0lb
10st 7lb	<7lb	7lb – 1st 1lb	>1st 1lb
10st 11lb	<8lb	8lb – 1st 1lb	>1st 1lb
11st	<8lb	8lb – 1st 1lb	>1st 1lb
11st 4lb	<8lb	8lb – 1st 2lb	>1st 2lb
11st 7lb	<8lb	8lb – 1st 2lb	>1st 2lb
11st 11lb	<8lb	8lb – 1st 3lb	>1st 3lb
12st	<8lb	8lb – 1st 3lb	>1st 3lb
12st 4lb	<9lb	9lb – 1st 3lb	>1st 3lb
12st 7lb	<9lb	9lb – 1st 4lb	>1st 4lb
12st 11lb	<9lb	9lb – 1st 4lb	>1st 4lb
13st	<9lb	9lb – 1st 4lb	>1st 4lb
13st 4lb	<9lb	9lb – 1st 5lb	>1st 5lb
13st 7lb	<9lb	9lb – 1st 5lb	>1st 5lb
13st 11lb	<10lb	10lb – 1st 5lb	>1st 5lb
14st	<10lb	10lb – 1st 6lb	>1st 6lb
14st 4lb	<10lb	10lb – 1st 6lb	>1st 6lb
14st 7lb	<10lb	10lb – 1st 6lb	>1st 6lb
14st 11lb	<10lb	10lb – 1st 7lb	>1st 7lb
15st	<11lb	11lb – 1st 7lb	>1st 7lb
15st 4lb	<11lb	11lb – 1st 7lb	>1st 7lb
15st 7lb	<11lb	11lb – 1st 8lb	>1st 8lb
15st 11lb	<11lb	11lb – 1st 8lb	>1st 8lb
16st	<11lb	11lb – 1st 8lb	>1st 8lb
16st 4lb	<11lb	11lb – 1st 9lb	>1st 9lb
16st 7lb	<12lb	12lb – 1st 9lb	>1st 9lb

© BAPEN

Alternative measurements and considerations

BAPEN
Advancing Clinical Nutrition
www.bapen.org.uk

Step 1: BMI (body mass index)

If height cannot be measured
- Use recently documented or self-reported height (if reliable and realistic).
- If the subject does not know or is unable to report their height, use one of the alternative measurements to estimate height (ulna, knee height or demispan).

Step 2: Recent unplanned weight loss

If recent weight loss cannot be calculated, use self-reported weight loss (if reliable and realistic).

Subjective criteria

If height, weight or BMI cannot be obtained, the following criteria which relate to them can assist your professional judgement of the subject's nutritional risk category. Please note, these criteria should be used collectively not separately as alternatives to steps 1 and 2 of 'MUST' and are not designed to assign a score. Mid upper arm circumference (MUAC) may be used to estimate BMI category in order to support your overall impression of the subject's nutritional risk.

1. BMI
- Clinical impression – thin, acceptable weight, overweight. Obvious wasting (very thin) and obesity (very overweight) can also be noted.

2. Unplanned weight loss
- Clothes and/or jewellery have become loose fitting (weight loss).
- History of decreased food intake, reduced appetite or swallowing problems over 3-6 months and underlying disease or psycho-social/physical disabilities likely to cause weight loss.

3. Acute disease effect
- Acutely ill and no nutritional intake or likelihood of no intake for more than 5 days.

Further details on taking alternative measurements, special circumstances and subjective criteria can be found in *The 'MUST' Explanatory Booklet*. A copy can be downloaded at www.bapen.org.uk or purchased from the BAPEN office. The full evidence-base for 'MUST' is contained in *The 'MUST' Report* and is also available for purchase from the BAPEN office.

BAPEN Office, Secure Hold Business Centre, Studley Road, Redditch, Worcs, B98 7LG. Tel: 01527 457 850. Fax: 01527 458 718. bapen@sovereignconference.co.uk   BAPEN is registered charity number 1023927.   www.bapen.org.uk

Royal College
of Nursing

© BAPEN. First published May 2004 by MAG the Malnutrition Advisory Group, a Standing Committee of BAPEN.
Reviewed and reprinted with minor changes March 2008 and September 2010
'MUST' is supported by the British Dietetic Association, the Royal College of Nursing and the Registered Nursing Home Association.

© BAPEN

Alternative measurements: instructions and tables

BAPEN
Advancing Clinical Nutrition
www.bapen.org.uk

If height cannot be obtained, use length of forearm (ulna) to calculate height using tables below.
(See The 'MUST' Explanatory Booklet for details of other alternative measurements (knee height and demispan) that can also be used to estimate height).

Estimating height from ulna length

Measure between the point of the elbow (olecranon process) and the midpoint of the prominent bone of the wrist (styloid process) (left side if possible).

HEIGHT (m) Men(<65years)	1.94	1.93	1.91	1.89	1.87	1.85	1.84	1.82	1.80	1.78	1.76	1.75	1.73	1.71
Men(≥65years)	1.87	1.86	1.84	1.82	1.81	1.79	1.78	1.76	1.75	1.73	1.71	1.70	1.68	1.67
Ulna length(cm)	32.0	31.5	31.0	30.5	30.0	29.5	29.0	28.5	28.0	27.5	27.0	26.5	26.0	25.5
HEIGHT (m) Women(<65years)	1.84	1.83	1.81	1.80	1.79	1.77	1.76	1.75	1.73	1.72	1.70	1.69	1.68	1.66
Women(≥65years)	1.84	1.83	1.81	1.79	1.78	1.76	1.75	1.73	1.71	1.70	1.68	1.66	1.65	1.63
HEIGHT (m) Men(<65years)	1.69	1.67	1.66	1.64	1.62	1.60	1.58	1.57	1.55	1.53	1.51	1.49	1.48	1.46
Men(≥65years)	1.65	1.63	1.62	1.60	1.59	1.57	1.56	1.54	1.52	1.51	1.49	1.48	1.46	1.45
Ulna length(cm)	25.0	24.5	24.0	23.5	23.0	22.5	22.0	21.5	21.0	20.5	20.0	19.5	19.0	18.5
HEIGHT (m) Women(<65years)	1.65	1.63	1.62	1.61	1.59	1.58	1.56	1.55	1.54	1.52	1.51	1.50	1.48	1.47
Women(≥65years)	1.61	1.60	1.58	1.56	1.55	1.53	1.52	1.50	1.48	1.47	1.45	1.44	1.42	1.40

Estimating BMI category from mid upper arm circumference (MUAC)

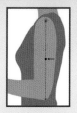

The subject's left arm should be bent at the elbow at a 90 degree angle, with the upper arm held parallel to the side of the body. Measure the distance between the bony protrusion on the shoulder (acromion) and the point of the elbow (olecranon process). Mark the mid-point.

Ask the subject to let arm hang loose and measure around the upper arm at the mid-point, making sure that the tape measure is snug but not tight.

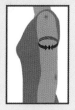

If MUAC is <23.5 cm, BMI is likely to be <20 kg/m².
If MUAC is >32.0 cm, BMI is likely to be >30 kg/m².

The use of MUAC provides a general indication of BMI and is not designed to generate an actual score for use with 'MUST'. For further information on use of MUAC please refer to *The 'MUST' Explanatory Booklet.*

© BAPEN

Source: the Malnutrition Universal Screening Tool (MUST) is reproduced here with the kind permission of BAPEN (British Association for Parenteral and Enteral Nutrition). For further information on MUST see www.bapen.org.uk

Appendix 3

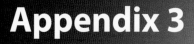

NATIONAL EARLY WARNING SCORE (NEWS 2) OBSERVATION CHART

Calculation Skills for Nurses, Second Edition. Claire Boyd.
© 2022 John Wiley & Sons Ltd. Published 2022 by John Wiley & Sons Ltd.

NEWS key

| 0 | 1 | 2 | 3 |

		DATE															DATE	
		TIME															TIME	

A+B Respirations Breaths/min	≥25									3					≥25
	21-24									2					21-24
	18-20														18-20
	15-17														15-17
	12-14														12-14
	9-11									1					9-11
	≤8									3					≤8

A+B SpO₂ Scale 1 Oxygen saturation (%)	≥96														≥96
	94-95									1					94-95
	92-93									2					92-93
	≤91									3					≤91

SpO₂ Scale 2† Oxygen saturation (%) Use Scale 2 if target range is 88-92%, e.g. in hypercapnic respiratory failure	≥97 on O₂									3					≥97 on O₂
	95-96 on O₂									2					95-96 on O₂
	93-94 on O₂									1					93-94 on O₂
↑ ONLY use Scale 2 under the direction of a doctor or the respiratory team	≥93 on air														≥93 on air
	88-92														88-92
	86-87														86-87
	84-85									2					84-85
	≤83%									3					≤83%

Air or oxygen?	A = Air														A = Air
	O₂ L/min									2					O₂ L/min
	Device														Device

C Blood Pressure mmHg Score uses systolic BP only	≥220									3					≥220
	201-219														201-219
	181-200														181-200
	161-180														161-180
	141-160														141-160
	121-140														121-140
	111-120														111-120
	101-110									1					101-110
	91-100									2					91-100
	81-90														81-90
	71-80									3					71-80
	61-70														61-70
	51-60														51-60
	≤50														≤50

C Pulse Beats/min	≥131									3					≥131
	121-130									2					121-130
	111-120														111-120
	101-110									1					101-110
	91-100														91-100
	81-90														81-90
	71-80														71-80
	61-70														61-70
	51-60														51-60
	41-50									1					41-50
	31-40									3					31-40
	≤30														≤30

D Consciousness Score for NEW onset of confusion (no score if chronic)	Alert														Alert
	New confusion														New confusion
	V									3					V
	P														P
	U														U

E Temperature °C	≥39.1°									2					≥39.1°
	38.1-39.0°									1					38.1-39.0°
	37.1-38.0°														37.1-38.0°
	36.1-37.0°														36.1-37.0°
	35.1-36.0°									1					35.1-36.0°
	≤35.0°									3					≤35.0°

NEWS2 Score															Score
Monitoring frequency															frequency
Escalation required? Y/N															Escalation
Pain score at rest															Pain rest
Pain score on moving															Pain moving
Pain score in use V or A (V=VAS, A- Abbey)															VAS, or Abbey
Nausea score															Nausea
Pruritis Score															Pruritis
Sedation Score															Sedation
Practitioner Initials															Initials
RN check per shift															RN check

Royal College of Physicians. National Early Warning Score (NEWS) 2: Standardising the assessment of acute-illness severity in the NHS. Updated report of a working party. London. RCP 2017

Appendix 4
· · · · · · · · · · · · · · · · · ·
WATERLOW PRESSURE ULCER PREVENTION/ TREATMENT POLICY

Calculation Skills for Nurses, Second Edition. Claire Boyd.
© 2022 John Wiley & Sons Ltd. Published 2022 by John Wiley & Sons Ltd.

WATERLOW PRESSURE ULCER PREVENTION/TREATMENT POLICY
RING SCORES IN TABLE, ADD TOTAL. MORE THAN 1 SCORE/CATEGORY CAN BE USED

BUILD/WEIGHT FOR HEIGHT		SKIN TYPE VISUAL RISK AREAS		SEX AGE		MALNUTRITION SCREENING TOOL (MST) (Nutrition Vol.15, No.6 1999 - Australia)		
AVERAGE BMI= 20-24.9	0	HEALTHY	0	MALE	1	A - HAS PATIENT LOST WEIGHT RECENTLY?	B - WEIGHT LOSS SCORE	
ABOVE AVERAGE BMI (25-29.9)	1	TISSUE PAPER	1	FEMALE	2	YES -GO TO B	0.5-5kg	= 1
OBESE BMI > 30	2	DRY	1	14-49	1	NO -GO TO C	5-10kg	= 2
BELOW AVERAGE BMI > 20	3	OEDEMATOUS	1	50-64	2	UNSURE - GO TO C AND SCORE 2	10-15kg	= 3
BMI = Wt(kg)/ Ht (m)^2		CLAMMY, PYREXIA	1	65-74	3		> 15kg	= 4
		DISCOLOURED GRADE 1	2	75-80	4		unsure	= 2
		BROKEN/SPOTS GRADE 2-4	3	81 +	5	C- PATIENT EATING POORLY /LACK OF APPETITE "NO"- 0; "YES" SCORE - 1	NUTRITION SCORE If > 2 refer for nutrition assessment / intervention	

CONTINENCE		MOBILITY		SPECIAL RISKS			
COMPLETE/ CATHETERISED	0	FULLY	0	TISSUE MALNUTRITION		NEUROLOGICAL DEFICIT	
URINE INCONT.	1	RESTLESS/FIDGETY	1	TERMINAL CACHEXIA	8	DIABETES, MS, CVA	4-6
FAECAL INCONT.	2	APATHETIC	2	MULTIPLE ORGAN FAILURE	8	MOTOR SENSORY	4-6
URINARY+ FAECAL INCONTINENCE	3	RESTRICTED	3	SINGLE ORGAN FAILURE (RESP, RENAL, CARDIAC)	5	PARAPLEGIA (MAX OF 6)	4-6
		BEDBOUND e.g. TRACTION	4	PERIPHERAL VASCULAR DISEASE	5	MAJOR SURGERY or TRAUMA	
		CHAIR BOUND e.g. WHEELCHAIR	5	ANAEMIA (Hb < 8)	2	ORTHOPAEDIC/SPINAL	5
				SMOKING	1	ON TABLE > 2 HR#	5
						ON TABLE > 6 HR#	8

MEDICATION - CYTOTOXICS LONG TERM/HIGH DOSE STEROIDS, ANTI-INFLAMMATORY   MAX OF 4

SCORE
10+ AT RISK
15+ HIGH RISK
20+ VERY HIGH RISK

© J Waterlow, Waterlow Score, 1985.
Obtainable from the Nook, Stoke Road, Henlade TAUNTON TA3 5LX
* The 2005 revision incorporates the research undertaken by Queensland Health.
www.judy-waterlow.co.uk
Scores can be discounted after 48 hours provided patient is recovering normally

Appendix 5
CONVERSION TABLES

KILOGRAMS TO POUNDS

1 kg = 2.2 lb

kg	lb	kg	lb	kg	lb	kg	lb	kg	lb	kg	lb
1	2.2	21	46.2	41	90.2	61	134.2	81	178.2	101	222.2
2	4.4	22	48.4	42	92.4	62	136.4	82	180.4	102	224.4
3	6.6	23	50.6	43	94.6	63	138.6	83	182.6	103	226.6
4	8.8	24	52.8	44	96.8	64	140.8	84	184.8	104	228.8
5	1.0	25	55.0	45	99.0	65	143.0	85	187.0	105	231.0
6	13.2	26	57.2	46	101.2	66	145.2	85	189.2	106	233.3
7	15.4	27	59.4	47	103.4	67	147.4	87	191.4	107	235.4
8	17.6	28	61.6	48	105.6	68	149.6	88	193.6	108	237.6
9	19.8	29	63.8	49	107.8	69	151.8	89	195.8	109	239.8
10	22.0	30	66.0	50	110.0	70	154.0	90	198.0	110	242.0
11	24.2	31	68.2	51	112.2	71	156.2	91	200.2	111	244.2
12	26.4	32	70.4	52	114.4	72	158.4	92	202.4	112	246.4
13	28.6	33	72.6	53	116.6	73	160.6	93	204.6	113	248.6
14	30.8	34	74.8	54	118.8	74	162.8	94	206.8	114	250.8
15	33.0	35	77.0	55	121.0	75	165.0	95	209.0	115	253.0
16	35.2	36	79.2	56	123.2	76	167.2	96	211.2	116	255.2
17	37.4	37	81.4	57	125.4	77	169.4	97	213.4	117	257.4
18	39.6	38	83.6	58	127.6	78	171.6	98	215.6	118	259.6
19	41.8	39	85.8	59	129.8	79	173.8	99	217.8	119	261.8
20	44.0	40	88.0	60	132.0	80	176.0	100	220.0	120	264.0

STONES TO KILOGRAMS

1 stone = 6.35 kg

stones	kg	stones	kg
1	6.35	15	95.25
2	12.7	16	101.6
3	19.05	17	107.95
4	25.4	18	114.3
5	31.75	19	120.65
6	38.1	20	127.0
7	44.45	21	133.35
8	50.8	22	139.7
9	57.15	23	146.05
10	63.5	24	152.4
11	69.85	25	158.75
12	76.2	26	165.1
13	82.55	27	171.45
14	88.9	28	177.8

POUNDS TO KILOGRAMS

1 lb = 0.45 kg

lb	kg
1	0.45
2	0.9
3	1.35
4	1.8
5	2.25
6	2.7
7	3.15
8	3.6
9	4.05
10	4.5
11	4.95
12	5.4
13	5.85
14 (1 stone)	6.35

HEIGHT CONVERSION CHART

Height (Feet and Inches)	Height (Inches)	Height (Metres)	Height (Centimetres)
4'	48	1.22	122
4'1"	49	1.24	124
4'2"	50	1.27	127
4'3"	51	1.29	129
4'4"	52	1.32	132
4'5"	53	1.35	135
4'6"	54	1.37	137
4'7"	55	1.4	140
4'8"	56	1.42	142
4'9"	57	1.45	145
4'10"	58	1.47	147
4'11"	59	1.5	150
5'	60	1.52	152
5'1"	61	1.55	155
5'2"	62	1.57	157
5'3"	63	1.6	160
5'4"	64	1.62	162
5'5"	65	1.65	165
5'6"	66	1.68	168
5'7"	67	1.7	170
5'8"	68	1.73	173
5'9"	69	1.75	175
5'10"	70	1.78	179
5'11"	71	1.8	180
6'	72	1.83	183
6'1"	73	1.85	185
6'2"	74	1.88	188
6'3"	75	1.9	190
6'4"	76	1.93	193

Converted to the nearest centimetre

USEFUL CONVERSIONS

1 kg = 2.2 lb
1 stone = 6.35 kg
1 lb = 0.45 kg
1 inch = 2.54 centimetres

Index

Calculation Skills for Nurses, Second Edition. Claire Boyd.
© 2022 John Wiley & Sons Ltd. Published 2022 by John Wiley & Sons Ltd.

INDEX